C000151582

Modern Strategy
for Preclinical
Pharmaceutical R&D

Modern Strategy for Preclinical Pharmaceutical R&D

Towards the Virtual Research Company

DAVID CAVALLA
Arachnova Ltd, Cambridge, UK

With contributions from
JOHN FLACK
AMRAD Corporation, Richmond, Australia
and
RICHARD JENNINGS
Wolfson Industrial Liaison Office, University of Cambridge, UK

JOHN WILEY & SONS
Chichester • New York • Weinheim • Brisbane • Singapore • Toronto

Copyright © 1997 John Wiley & Sons Ltd,
Baffins Lane, Chichester,
West Sussex PO19 1UD, England

National   01243 779777
International (+44) 1243 779777
e-mail (for orders and customer service enquiries):
cs-books@wiley.co.uk
Visit our Home Page on http://www.wiley.co.uk
or http://www.wiley.com

Reprinted October 1999

All rights reserved. No part of this publication may be reproduced, stored in a retrieval
system, or transmitted, in any form or by any means, electronic, mechanical, photocopying,
recording, scanning or otherwise, except under the terms of the Copyright, Designs and
Patents Act 1988 or under the terms of a licence issued by the Copyright Licensing Agency,
90 Tottenham Court Road, London, UK W1P 9HE, without the permission in writing of
the publisher.

Other Wiley Editorial Offices

John Wiley & Sons, Inc., 605 Third Avenue,
New York, NY 10158-0012, USA

VCH Verlagsgesellschaft mbH, Pappelallee 3,
D-69469 Weinheim, Germany

Jacaranda Wiley Ltd, 33 Park Road, Milton,
Queensland 4064, Australia

John Wiley & Sons (Asia) Pte Ltd, 2 Clementi Loop #02-01,
Jin Xing Distripark, Singapore 129809

John Wiley & Sons (Canada) Ltd, 22 Worcester Road,
Rexdale, Ontario M9W 1L1, Canada

Library of Congress Cataloging-in-Publication Data

Cavalla, David.
    Modern strategy for preclinical pharmaceutical R&D : towards the virtual research
company / David Cavalla ; with contributions from John Flack and Richard Jennings.
       p.   cm.
    Includes bibliographical references and index.
    ISBN 0-471-97117-0 (hbk. : alk. paper)
    1. Drugs—Research—Management.   2. Pharmaceutical industry.
3. Drugs—Research—Economic aspects.   I. Flack, John D.
II. Jennings, Richard, 1948–   .   III. Title.
    [DNLM: 1. Drug Industry—organization & administration.
2. Drug Industry—economics.   3. Research Design.   QV 736 C377m 1997]
RM301.25.C38 1997
615'.19—dc21
DNLM/DLC
for Library of Congress   96-37234
                                                                        CIP

British Library Cataloguing in Publication Data

A catalogue record for this book is available from the British Library

ISBN 0-471-97117-0

Typeset in 10/12pt Palatino from author's disks by Mayhew Typesetting, Rhayader, Powys
Printed and bound in Great Britain

This book is printed on acid-free paper responsibly manufactured from sustainable
forestation, for which at least two trees are planted for each one used for paper production.

Contents

Preface

If, as a new entrant to the pharmaceutical industry, you have picked up this book and are wondering if modern strategy is a concern solely for the chiefs and not the Indians, consider this. The question of how, when, where and if to conduct pharmaceutical research has profound implications, not just for those in the industry itself. Academia is increasingly dependent on industrial sources of funding for research, but this support is not one way, since the industry too is reliant on the ability of these institutions to supply qualified scientists to it. Moreover, the decision to close a pharmaceutical research centre has implications both for the economy and for the wider science and technology base of its national location. The prognosis is for further such closures and emergence of small companies too. Scientists are well known for ignoring their surroundings while concentrating on their work, but if you can hear the low rumble of a distant storm, shouldn't you at least check the wind direction?

This book arose from my work at Napp together with a feeling that the present view of pharmaceutical research and development is based with an eye to the past, rather than the future. The twentieth century has been a great success for modern medicine, and has resulted in the generation of many drugs to treat most common illnesses. However, there is a tendency to leave it at that, with no attempt to confront critics of the industry who, for a variety of reasons, object to the concept of obtaining profit from human illness, or to examine the profound changes which have occurred as a result of recent mergers, acquisitions and consolidations. My feeling was that some order among the chaos would be beneficial, even if only to manage the future.

The heart of the question is to determine whether the economies of scale arising from the increasing size of the large multinational pharmaceutical companies adequately compensate for the loss of creative individualism that is essential for the process of drug discovery and development. Conversely, it is to determine whether technological experts might better provide services to a number of clients rather than work within a single large infrastructure where confidentiality is paramount, and synergy of multidisciplinary operation rarely possible. The complexity of new product introduction in pharmaceuticals, the level of risk and of investment, demand enquiry as to whether there might be a better way.

This book attempts to answer these questions by exploring the advantages and disadvantages of collaborative methods of drug research, and whether in the extreme, it may be possible to arrive at the so-called virtual research company, which does no practical work itself but merely co-ordinates the work of others. For those who are familiar with the economics of pharmaceutical R&D, the suggestions for reduced development costs made by these stratagems must draw serious analysis.

I should like to thank those who have helped in the production of this book, some directly through discussions over the years and through encouragement, others indirectly in having read and commented on the unfinished form. In particular, I would like to thank: my father, Dr John Cavalla, for assistance in both these areas; Dr Hank Agersborg who deserves credit for his contributions from his own experience to making this book both more coherent and inclusive; Drs John Flack and Richard Jennings who, in addition to contributing significantly to the text of the publication, supported its philosophical purpose as a commentary on modern drug research and development from an early stage; and last, but not least, Dr Louise Milne for her erudite advice on the art and architecture of the flying buttress.

Cambridge, August 1996

Introduction

There is an ongoing debate about the correct response to the intensifying pressures, relating to the increasing costs of new products, and the decreasing returns besetting the pharmaceutical industry. At the heart of this debate is the question of whether there should be increasingly large vertically integrated transnational corporations doing all that is necessary to bring products to market. This includes researching, developing, registering, marketing, selling and conducting all the other ancillary tasks, including patient health management, necessary in the business of pharmaceuticals. As an alternative, some of these functions could be broken up and performed by specialist companies. Many believe that there is an increasing place for such specialist companies that can offer niche services to a number of clients, working in partnership with multinational pharmaceutical companies who alone possess the global marketing presence to maximise the sales return to R&D investment.

Research and development in the industry has been one of the functions most hard hit by the recent changes, and the effect has been twofold. On the one hand, as large pharmaceutical multinationals have reduced their internal research activities there has been a huge spawning of many varied start-up companies. On the other hand, there has been an increasing reliance on contracted research in an effort to increase flexibility. Both of these measures have increased cost-awareness and cost-responsibility in drug research. To a certain extent, the present revolution is merely a belated response to the increasing costs of pharmaceutical research and development, which in the years 1981 to 1992 rose globally from a little over $5bn to around $22bn.[1] This rise, which has brought the average spend on pharmaceutical R&D to around 15% of revenues, was brought about by a number of factors:

- increasingly difficult regulatory environments fed by public concern about safety
- increasingly onerous clinical studies to prove efficacy
- need to conduct investigations into cost-effectiveness of new medicines
- greatest financial reward lying in increasingly difficult therapeutic categories
- greater cost of laboratory equipment, personnel, standards of laboratory health and safety

In addition to the increased difficulty in bringing new products to the market, there have been financial pressures on the industry from loss of revenue, brought about by:

- more efficient generic competition and therapeutic substitution
- greater pressure on reimbursement prices, which need to be justified by pharmacoeconomics
- loss of effective patent-protected life

The threat from generic competition has been particularly pronounced because of the number of major drugs that have lost or will be losing patent protection in the 1990s. Some companies have considered it apposite to involve themselves in managed care and pharmacy benefit management companies, beyond the mere provision of pharmaceutical products. Others have taken the view that R&D is fundamental to both the current operation and future prospects of the industry, but that a grassroots analysis of the direction and efficiency of the processes by which new products are to be created is necessary.

The current penchant for alternatives to large pharmaceutical R&D is partly a herd-like reaction to a perceived need to change the traditional approach. The upheaval of the past few years has brought, in many cases, a muddled response. There is little doubt that the industry of today is little like that of 20 or even 10 years ago. Under these circumstances, there is a feeling that the wisdom of experience may count for little. Early retirement and downsizing have rid the industry of many of its elder statesmen, but it has struggled to find coherence behind a single view of how to respond to today's agenda.

Amid the turmoil created by these pressures, fundamental questions on strategic plans of major pharmaceutical companies are being asked. In an effort to uncover new approaches, increasing reliance is being placed on the views of external consultants.[2] Many of these people have eminence in other fields, many with track records of success in other businesses. They compare the experiences in other areas such as the motor industry and computers, where problems of overcapacity and competition have brought about a culture of contractual relationships. Suppliers of component parts are sometimes quite large in themselves, but they have to react quickly to the needs of their clients, and provide top quality at the lowest cost.

The protectionist forces surrounding the patenting of inventions that bring up to 20 years of marketing exclusivity, even when eroded by at least 5–6 years of development time, create monopolies that are not found elsewhere. Unlike the case with many industries, the consumer does not exercise a direct choice on the product that he or she buys. The prescribing doctor exercises that choice, but rarely is there an incentive to make cost an overriding factor. In most countries, the payment for the prescription comes largely from government, and even in the US, where this is not the case, insurance funds most of the cost. Additional pressure is brought to bear these days by a number of other organisations, such as regulators, insurers, pressure groups and even (sometimes) the patients themselves. This is a strange market indeed, not easily modelled by economists. It is invidious to compare the pharmaceutical industry with these other examples, but some lessons can perhaps be brought across.

The mood of change brings great uncertainty. While it is now increasingly recognised that the best way forward is through improved medicines, the demands placed on the industry in terms of performance for these new entrants imply that the difficulties of discovering and developing them are commensurately greater. Given the uncertainty, given the difficulty of prediction, the investment in research and development activities comes in for much attention.

Pharmaceutical research and development is one of the most difficult problems of project management in any industry today, and is getting more difficult. It has been compared to a very complicated construction project, which would traditionally be done almost exclusively by contract. However, a significant extra dimension of complexity is afforded by the risk involved, and the lack of a guarantee that any commercial end-point will be reached. Perhaps the organisation of a Formula One racing team is a better analogy, given the time, expense, application and risk required for the winning of the annual Grand Prix trophy (see p. 82). Pharmaceutical development has been a focus for streamlining for some time, and in consequence a good deal of clinical development has been routinely conducted in the past in a contract setting. There is sound experience behind the success of these arrangements and good evidence that it works. But the track record in regard to extramural pharmaceutical research is patchy at best.

This environment is now changing: contract research organisations (CROs) are increasingly advertising their capability to be involved with discovery and early drug development, with an emphasis on partnership; a flurry of entrepreneurial activity is establishing a large number of small research-based companies intent on collaborating with larger partners; and universities are marketing their technological expertise for commercial gain. The appetite of larger companies for collaborative ventures is growing rapidly, and recent evidence suggests this trend will gather pace.

The dividing line between pharmaceutical research and development may be difficult to draw, but one thing is clear: the greatest risk attaches to the operations conducted nearer the start of a pharmaceutical project. In taking up the offer from external collaborators to assist at ever earlier stages in the process, large pharmaceutical companies are effectively asking for help in spreading this risk. And in making the offer, such collaborators may in many cases be taking on a bigger risk than they can comfortably handle.

The reasons for the trends towards outsourcing may lie in the accumulated pressures of the past, but a consideration of the future benefit suggests that this may become the preferred modality for the future of pharmaceutical research. The potential advantages apply to both the small and large pharmaceutical company, for both the academic and industrial sectors. Zeneca recently announced an increase in R&D spending to allow for more alliances with small technology providers. This is at a time when R&D spending is already at a historic high. So why is the spending increasing, and why is it focused on such companies?

One answer lies in the finances of drug research, and another in the revolution in drug discovery technology. Late stage research is expensive, and commands a large proportion of a company's R&D budget. To ensure only the best candidates are progressed through to market, a larger number of such candidates are required: candidates that will change the face of medicine, that are of 'breakthrough' quality and that will bring blockbuster returns. Calculations of the number of new drug applications (NDAs) that the major companies will need in future to support their massive R&D expenditures make sobering reading. Glaxo are hoping they can increase the output to the launch of three new chemical entities (NCEs) per year by the start of the next century. On the other hand, if the cost of drug development can be reduced to bare essentials, perhaps this ambitious goal may become more modest and easy to achieve. The figures that are perhaps possible if development can be fully outsourced suggest that the savings may be very real indeed.

At the other extreme, basic research has brought advances in molecular biology that will unravel the human genome, creating a huge haystack of DNA sequences within which the elusive needle of the blockbuster is hidden. This new technology has been complemented by the automation of other laboratory procedures, particularly the changes in synthetic chemistry brought by combinatorial techniques. Small-scale, pilot research across a much larger number of molecular targets is required to identify which targets are worthy of greatest attention, coupled with a more rigorous application of financial principles to determine what is progressed through to market. Contracted discovery and preclinical development can serve both of these requirements, and large companies are increasingly persuaded of this fact.

This book will start with a definition of the processes involved in drug discovery and development. The subsequent chapters 2 and 3 will address the advantages and disadvantages of collaborations in the context of the challenges presently facing the pharmaceutical industry. These will be written mainly from the viewpoint of the 'buyer' of the contract or collaboration, rather than the 'seller'; this is to reflect the fact that the greatest change in the situation has been from the large company attitude to these arrangements. The emphasis on discovery and the early stages of development will reflect the author's experience, but the philosophy behind outsourcing may also be held to be similar in later stages of pharmaceutical development. Chapters 4 and 5 will deal in detail with the roles that academia and industry can play as contractors and collaborative bodies in pharmaceutical R&D. The situation, especially with regard to the emergence of small multidisciplinary companies as research boutiques, is changing rapidly, and these chapters will deal with salient features of the present situation rather than attempt to include all the providers of such services. The purpose is to outline the scope of the possibilities, rather than include all those within the field. Every attempt has been made to ensure accuracy, but this cannot be guaranteed, especially in a situation that is changing so rapidly.

The types of collaboration vary considerably from that which is common with academia, to that with CROs, to that now being seen with small research companies. Many of the latter have been grouped by the term 'biotechnology' company, when the variation between them is too large, and the connection with biotechnology too tenuous, to make this adjective a useful one. In fact, such companies may have very different philosophical and strategic objectives, ranging from those that aim to specialise in a single discipline (the technology provider of, for instance, combinatorial chemistry) to those that offer complete research programmes. Furthermore, the stage at which collaborations are sought by these companies varies enormously, with some looking for partners almost at the outset of a project, and others waiting until some results from human administration, or even concerning clinical efficacy, are available.

The aim of this book is to examine in detail the reasons for the trend for partnerships and collaborations, and to determine what the potential advantages are to the modern pharmaceutical industry. What are the problems? What are the solutions? What are the long-term prognostications for this mode of research? And finally, chapter 6 will ask what is the logical end-point—how much if anything needs to occur in-house?

One purpose of this last section is to describe the structure, or architecture, of pharmaceutical R&D, to emphasise the interaction of different disciplines required to bring a drug to the market. The principles behind the collaborative potential of the academic, CRO and biotechnology sectors are quite different. The ways in which they can strategically interact with the traditional pharmaceutical industry, and increasingly with each other, are important to understand. New models by which the edifice of a drug R&D project can be constructed can be considered, including ones which bypass the large pharmaceutical company entirely, but which place increasing importance on the integrative capability of the virtual research company. Although small and emerging, such companies are quite distinct in philosophy from the rest of the biotechnology sector. Their involvement is as project management companies, who can function often without any laboratory work, and without the level of investment required by the research boutiques or even the single technology providers. If they are successful, and this is by no means clear at present, the finances of drug discovery and development may change considerably, permitting consideration of medicines for markets which are currently not thought to be sufficiently commercially attractive. We live in interesting times.

1
The Pharmaceutical
Development Process

Pharmaceutical companies need to invest hugely in research and development to survive. Before looking at ways in which this process may be made more efficient, it is appropriate to define what the pharmaceutical development process entails.

1.1 DEFINITION

The discovery and development of a new drug leading to registration and approval for human therapeutic use is conventionally divided into these stages:

- discovery research
- preclinical development
- clinical development
  ◇ Phase I
  ◇ Phase II
  ◇ Phase III

Discovery research produces an entity with the desired biological action. The aim of preclinical development is to garner sufficient information on the safety, ancillary pharmacology, disposition and side-effects following administration of the drug candidate to animals for progression into humans in Phase I. In the US, this process is regulated by the Food and Drug Administration (FDA), and consideration of an Investigational New Drug (IND) submission is required for these studies to commence. In the UK, there is no legal requirement of this sort, but an Ethics Committee needs to approve the study, and in practice the standards that are demanded are closely similar. Phases I through III involve human trials of increasing complexity. Phases II and III involve patients with the target disease or condition. The approval to market a new drug comes from submission of data after completion of Phase III studies. In the US, new drug applications (NDAs) are regulated and approved by the FDA.

Since Phase I evaluation involves administration to human volunteers, often without therapeutic assessment, its description as a *clinical* phase of development is open to debate. Many definitions of preclinical development therefore include Phase I human volunteer trials. In addition, some of the activities that conventionally take place prior to clinical trials also extend to time periods concurrent with such trials. This is most obviously the case for toxicology assessments, since the more long-term studies (carcinogenicity and to a certain extent teratology) will normally extend well into the clinical testing phase. Similarly, there may be elements of the chemical development or pharmaceutical development work which extend into the clinical phase. As will be explained later, the phasing of certain studies may be changed in order to address foreseeable problems as early as possible. This type of development, with an emphasis on conducting critical assessments early on, has been termed the 'fast-fail' method.[3]

Because of all the above complexities, the demarcation between preclinical and clinical development is not a sharp one. There are elements which span both phases, and elements which can shift backwards or forwards depending on the particular problems and needs of the project at hand. The overall process can take anywhere from 7 to 12 years, involving hundreds of scientists, and thousands or tens of thousands of patients before any commercial return can be considered. There are, however, therapeutic categories, such as AIDS treatment, where the need for effective therapy is sufficiently acute that product approval may be based on much shorter developmental times, and small clinical studies involving as few as 20 patients.

Various metaphors have been used to describe the process of pharmaceutical drug discovery and development. Each emphasises one or more parts of the process, but is incomplete on its own. Examples of these metaphors include a horse-race, a poker game (both emphasising risk), a hurdles-race and an orchestra (emphasising organisational complexity). These are more fully described in Bert Spilker's treatise on *Drug Discovery and Development*.[4] Time and cost savings in the development process are obvious items for consideration in the current commercial climate. However, many companies have also focused their review on the preclinical stage of research and development because the choice of drug candidate for subsequent progression is critical.

The first two stages of drug discovery are taken to include the stages of basic research involving at least medicinal chemistry and biology (and maybe other disciplines) together with initial toxicological, metabolic and analytical studies required for entry into human volunteers.

1.2 PRECLINICAL RESEARCH

The traditional research process may be broken down into the following steps/activities:

- proposal of research project and assembly of project team
- synthesis of drug candidates
- biological evaluation *in vitro*
- biological evaluation *in vivo*

This is followed in the preclinical development phase by examination of metabolism and toxicology, and of physical properties related to the suitability of the chemical for administration to humans as a medicament.

1.2.1 Research proposal

Arguably the most crucial decision, and one that will ultimately vitally affect the chances of success in pharmaceutical R&D, comes right at the beginning. A hypothesis is made, generally along the lines that interaction in a particular biochemical mechanism will result in therapeutic benefit. The evidence is usually sketchy, the probability that the hypothesis is correct is far less than 100%. This is particularly the case with many of the multicomponent, multifaceted targets considered now by the industry. Modern pharmaceutical R&D is hampered greatly by its prior success: the ability to treat many common ailments with a reasonable degree of satisfaction now offers little enticement for new approaches to these diseases. The therapeutic targets that remain are significantly more challenging than many of those pursued even 15 years ago, but this fact has not been registered in the public's attitude to the drug industry.

Partly because of such increased difficulty, partly because of enhanced standards and requirements for safety, the costs of bringing new products to market have increased substantially. This has been amply dealt with in other writings (see section 1.4 and section 2.1); as a result, the potential rewards from research proposals are scrutinised in detail. Therapeutic entities with marketing projections less than $150m a year are rarely considered viable by major pharmaceutical companies with large sales forces to detail. Niche players do consider smaller markets, but try to do so without the requirement for full-blown new chemical entity programmes. Such approaches include biologically derived products, because of the greater degree of certainty (i.e. lesser uncertainty) surrounding that development passage. However, it should also be borne in mind that the cost of manufacture for early toxicological evaluation and clinical trials is a significant disincentive to the biotechnological approach. Other approaches also include novel drug delivery technologies, which can dramatically increase the appeal of an already registered chemical entity without the burden of much of the safety assessment, or exposure to horrendous adverse risk.

New chemical entities nevertheless remain the mainstay of most pharmaceutical research, because, by and large, organic molecules with molecular weights below 500 are those most likely to possess the capacity to provide blockbuster drugs of the next century.

Certain proposals can be made on evidence of a clinical kind, that supports the hypothetical role of a particular biochemical pathway in a human disease. There may be existing therapies which could derive substantial benefit from removal of side-effects associated with extraneous actions at unwanted sites. An example of this was the discovery by Glaxo of sumatriptan, based on the hypothesis that ergotamine derived its benefit in migraine from an ability to constrict the vasculature of the carotid bed. Glaxo were able, through an extensive medicinal chemistry programme, to enhance the carotid-selective actions of a series of new drugs, while minimising effects on other vascular beds. The result of this project was sumatriptan, a ground-breaking product for the treatment of migraine, and vastly superior to its antecedent ergotamine in terms of side-effects. This is an example of a hypothesis targeted towards reducing side-effects of an existing, therapeutically effective treatment.

Another example of a hypothesis leading to therapy is in the area of cholesterol-lowering agents. High cholesterol, or hypercholesterolemia, is a major dependent risk factor linked to increased mortality due to myocardial infarction. Since cholesterol enters the body pool from only two sources, diet or endogenous synthesis, one of the routes to tackling hypercholesterolemia was thought to be by inhibition of the major rate-limiting enzyme of such synthesis. This enzyme, HMG-CoA reductase, was found to be inhibited by a fungal metabolite, lovastatin, and this molecule went on to become the first approved treatment for primary hypercholesterolemia with this biochemical mode of action, effective in 30–50% of patients in lowering both total and low-density lipoprotein cholesterol. Subsequent synthetic improvements provided more potent molecules, and this class of molecule now provides a substantial element of therapy for this condition, although there remain side-effects including gastro-intestinal disorders, myopathy and increased liver enzymes.

Research in the pharmaceutical industry is sufficiently competitive that inevitably more than one company follows a particular approach. Analysis of the market need for a particular approach, or scientific validity thereof, is often based on publicly available data, to which every company has access. Historically, it has been possible to base research proposals on modes of action that are clinically proven to be effective, or even in some cases have reached the market. Such 'me-too' approaches were very common in, for instance, the β-blocker therapy of hypertension and cyclooxygenase inhibition for pain (NSAIDs—non-steroidal anti-inflammatory drugs). Current and future research projects are unlikely to have the luxury of this foreknowledge. Governments in the major pharmaceutical markets are reluctant to offer the commercial framework for such late entrants to the market to succeed, and review by the regulatory authorities is likely to include the requirement for real medical advantage over existing treatments. The current competitive climate in the industry can often result in a certain approach becoming favoured and adopted by half a dozen or more groups, without a clinical mandate having been produced. Companies who wish to move quickly need to have some ongoing research interests in the field, in order to be able to take on a project as rapidly as possible once the scientific evidence becomes sufficiently compelling. Thus, for example, the endothelin antagonists have been a popular target for anti-inflammatory and anti-thrombotic drugs; more specific versions of NSAIDs, which are thought to possess the beneficial but not the gastric side-effects of these therapeutic agents for arthritic and other inflammatory diseases, are also the subject of multiple groups' research. The theoretical basis for these research proposals comes from an understanding of the disease mechanisms and pharmacology of animal models: the validation of the theory in a human setting will come too late for new projects to be started, there will simply be too many others ahead in the field. Those that have yet to embark may merely sit and hope that their scepticism will have been well founded.

1.2.2   Chemistry

The goal of the medicinal chemistry team is to synthesise compounds for primary biological evaluation (screening) and, based on the results, to optimise the potency and other characteristics to achieve a lead drug candidate for further development. The process will involve, typically, the synthesis of hundreds or thousands of target molecules before a lead is selected. In addition to newly synthesised compounds, the vast libraries available to large pharmaceutical companies from historic projects may be trawled for lead discovery. Indeed, there are several possible approaches to the discovery of chemical leads described, rather cynically, by Dr J Babiak (Wyeth-Ayerst, Princeton, NJ) as belonging to one of a number of traits:

- serendipity (luck)
- random screening (dumb luck)
- copying someone else's patent (bad luck)
- copying someone else's drug (very bad luck)

This is a little prejudiced. Cox describes the research process as a mixture of serendipity and structured research.[5] It is fairer to describe the identification of medicinal chemical targets as based on an iterative feedback process resulting from the data produced by biological evaluation. The efficiency of the research is governed by the rapidity of the feedback process. In addition to the potency of the drug candidate, one of the key parameters, which is normally assessed by biochemical techniques, is that of a compound's selectivity. The biochemical multiplicity of receptors and enzymes has created increasingly high expectations and requirements for new drugs in this respect. The medicinal chemist seeks potency and selectivity for a lead candidate in the desired receptor assay; but as the number of known receptors increases, the demands of selectivity become harder to meet. The old-fashioned approach based on more empirical animal models, many of them *in vivo* models, may have permitted a less stringent biochemical selectivity, while simultaneously offering an early assessment of drug bioavailability which is often now only evaluated at a later stage in the discovery process.

Assembly of data from a number of similar compounds leads to production of structure–activity relationships for which quantitative methods of evaluation are possible (QSAR).[6] In their purest form, rational methods of drug design involve interpretation of a known biomolecular structure, and knowledge of an enzyme's or receptor's active site.[7] The improved ability to study ligand–receptor complexes by X-ray diffraction has been an important new development that has fortified the concept of structure-based drug design. This method involves analysis of the structure of the target biomolecule and sometimes of the ligand–target complex, which is often followed by computational techniques to design improved molecules for further synthesis. Qualitative interpretation is coupled with iterative cycles of biological assessment in the normal way, but the incorporation of physical techniques and molecular modelling gives an improved understanding of the basis for potency, and enhances the medicinal chemist's ability to design more potent ligands.

In addition to X-ray crystallographic techniques, more sophisticated methods of n.m.r. analysis have been used to measure 3-dimensional structure. Naturally, the X-ray methods are representative of a solid-state environment, which may differ from the solution phase in which biological interactions occur. Furthermore, the mere interaction of ligand with biomolecule still leaves a number of significant problems for the medicinal chemist to tackle. For example, information on one of the most widely studied enzymes, renin, is available from the related protein, pepsin; programmes to discover renin inhibitors have made substantial use of this information in an effort to rationally design useful drugs. However, concrete examples where such infor-mation has led directly to a clinically effective therapy are difficult to find; saquinavir, a specific protease inhibitor of the virus found in HIV, is one of them. But in others, such as in the case of renin, the major problems lay not with the design of potent inhibitors, but in the achievement of satisfactory bioavailability and resolution of other pharmaceutical problems, such as rapid biliary excretion. While progress has been made in this regard, these problems have not been solved and no renin inhibitor has yet reached the market.[8]

Scientific discovery along rational lines is fascinating and intensely motivating for any medicinal chemist. But the problems with renin inhibitors exemplify a principle that the objective of the chemist has in many cases remained the same, to produce a small molecule capable of crossing biological membranes to intervene in a biological process. Such a goal, requiring the identification of the part of the large (often proteinaceous) mediator that must be mimicked or blocked, is a ferociously difficult process. By comparison, modifica-tion of a small non-peptide neurotransmitter such as adrenaline (epinephrine) is straightforward. The means by which a fairly large peptide such as endothelin can be impeded at its binding site by molecules 10–20% of its size are difficult to understand, let alone predict by computer techniques.

Drug discovery owes a great deal to the chemical diversity of nature for the production of leads. Natural product screening programmes have historically been a significant part of the process of lead production, and a great many projects have begun from the basis of a natural product's activity in a certain assay. Over half of the current 25 best-selling drugs owe their discovery at least in part to natural products, and few will argue even today that this source can be ignored in lead generation. Most if not all pharmaceutical companies of any size have collections of plants and fungi from around the world, and routinely prepare extracts for testing. Current effort in this area is geared towards accelerated identification of new secondary metabolites, using techniques such as linked spectroscopic-chromatographic databases for the elimination of known compounds which may produce false positive 'hits'. Isolation and identification of new natural products employs automated chromatographic tools such as hplc-ms. However, the future for natural products may also include their use as templates for further elaboration in combinatorial chemistry programmes. The techniques for such elaboration may include traditional chemical as well as biochemical methods, and this possibility has been dubbed combinatorial biosynthesis.

Certain drugs have arisen from projects that have bypassed the medicinal chemist's input into design of small, usually non-peptidic, compounds. This approach applies particularly for many of the newer large molecule biological targets which are so very difficult to mimic by small molecules. Biotechnologically derived therapies are often peptides produced via molecular biological manipulation (see section 1.2.3). Such molecules do not normally lend themselves to oral administration, and are often designed to be given intravenously. Nevertheless, this approach clearly has delivered its successes with drugs such as Amgen's erythropoietin for anaemia, where intravenous administration is acceptable. There are many other examples of drugs in development aiming for therapy using recombinant proteins, that acknowledge the need for intravenous administration but expect to produce substantial returns.

The use of monoclonal antibodies directed against a natural peptide or protein is a particularly common approach to the interdiction of pathways that involve large intercellular messengers of this type. In addition to the problem of delivery, the main problem for monoclonal antibodies is the prevention of the body's natural immune reaction. This is especially so for chronic therapy, where the immune system can be expected to sensitise to the monoclonal on repeated dosing. A great deal of attention is paid to the assembly of monoclonals which have been humanised, to possess as much 'self' character as possible, which will diminish the processes of rejection.

One of the most revolutionary aspects of new drug discovery is the increasing adoption of robotic techniques and computerised methods of data handling and manipulation. Such automated methodology is actually composed of three parts, which together vastly expand the armoury of drug discovery:

- combinatorial synthesis
- high-throughput screening
- data handling

The powerful technique of combinatorial chemistry represents a new tool for medicinal chemists. In it, vast arrays of compounds are synthesised that can be assayed by high-throughput screening techniques. As described earlier, traditional synthesis techniques lead to the synthesis of individual compounds. Much store is placed on the purity of the products. Combinatorial chemistry turns traditional synthetic chemistry on its head: multiple, parallel syntheses without separation create libraries of compounds for testing. The purity of the products for testing is not a requirement; in fact, in some paradigms, impure products are positively required, since mixtures enhance the probability of success being achieved. The traditional manual techniques have been replaced by sophisticated automation. The principle of combinatorial chemistry involves the replacement of individual reactants by arrays of compounds. As shown in Figure 1.1, two N-membered arrays can give rise to N-squared possibilities in a single one-pot combinatorial reaction. As the number of reactions increases, the number of possible products increases exponentially. Thus, there are theoretically N^{S+1} products from a reaction sequence of S steps employing arrays (or basis sets) of N compounds.[9]

The methods of combinatorial chemistry differ substantially from traditional techniques. Although originally directed towards oligo-peptide or oligonucleotide synthesis, the interest is increasingly focusing on novel methods of making small non-peptide molecules as potential drugs capable of oral delivery. The synthetic methods often involve reactions on a solid phase support. The power of this technique makes expertise in this field extremely valuable to a pharmaceutical company.

Combinatorial chemistry has a potential impact on two areas of drug discovery:

- lead discovery
- lead optimisation

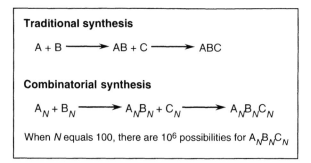

Figure 1.1   *Chemical equations in traditional and combinatorial organic synthesis*

Though there is a complementarity in terms of the technology used,[10] the strategy for each objective is different. Lead discovery, in which for instance a complicated large peptide is required to be mimicked by a small molecule, would require a large diverse set of structures to be investigated in the hope of finding a compound with modest but sufficient activity for optimisation. The second objective would require a relatively narrower set of structures to be investigated with the aim of maximising the potency and/or selectivity of the original lead.

   Diversity measurement is an important aspect of combinatorial chemistry. A successful mass-screening programme depends upon a library of varying molecular structure. For lead discovery, it is essential that the range of structures is wide but sufficiently complete to allow a reasonable degree of likelihood to be assumed that specific structural classes have been well analysed by the structures chosen. For lead optimisation, the range of structural types is necessarily narrower, although it needs to test the limits of the possibilities around the available lead. A variety of molecular characteristics, such as molecular weight, molar volume, calculated lipophilicity and dipole moment, as well as feature-to-feature distances have been used to quantify chemical diversity. Measuring diversity allows selection of a subset of samples that approximates the diversity of the whole library. A recent review of this subject reveals a number of approaches that have been used.[11] Another use of computerised techniques that is gaining increased prominence in drug discovery is based on the combination of molecular modelling and automated database searching of commercial collections of chemicals. Thus 3D database searching allows the chemist to select a set of compounds based on known active structures or from a knowledge of the binding site of a particular biomolecule.[12]

Closely allied to new combinatorial techniques of synthesis and the increased numbers of compounds for test, are robotic means of biological evaluation and data acquisition and analysis. Such techniques are being applied not just to compounds emanating from combinatorial chemistry programmes, but also from historic compound banks available in pharmaceutical company archives, and from natural sources.[13]

Two aspects of high-throughput screening relate to the protocol for initial screen and to the robotic techniques to enable its automation. The latter will not work properly without due attention to the former. Methods to optimise assay conditions given the numerous variables at play are important for the development of robotic screens. Both the theory and practice of assay design are themselves topics for discussion. Statistical experimental design is one approach to the development and optimisation of high-throughput screens.[14] The techniques are rapidly changing as the number of tests that are demanded increases exponentially. As assays are miniaturised, the use of radioactivity as a measure is being questioned, because of the time taken to achieve reliable estimates of ever smaller quantities of radioactivity, and alternative techniques are being considered. The move away from the traditional 96-well plate to the larger 384-well format and even beyond is well underway. Newer methods employing fluorescence techniques such as homogeneous time-resolved fluorescence (HTRF) are being developed for many applications. As far as the robotic techniques used in screening are concerned, it has been suggested that before implementation, one conducts a simulation of the process in order to verify what is expected to be produced.[15] Such a process allows the identification of potential bottlenecks, creation of 'what-if' scenarios and optimisation and quantification of the output.

In the race to adopt the new technologies, collaborative arrangements between large and small companies are the norm. This is dealt with in detail in sections 5.2.1.2 and 5.2.2.

1.2.3   Biology

The scientific method of drug discovery is organised around a tiered sequence of biological assays that are tied to the project. These assays, knowledge of which (and consideration of relevance to the disease process) usually forms part of the research proposal, are composed of a series of increasingly demanding tests to assess biological activity. An example, shown in Figure 1.2, begins with a biochemical screen to determine *in vitro* activity in a receptor binding or enzyme assay. Following demonstration of activity, it is common to undertake

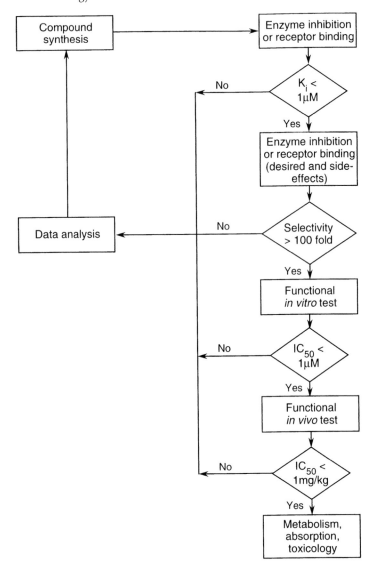

Figure 1.2   *An idealised project flow chart*

secondary biochemical assays to determine selectivity relative to other systems, and proceed with an assessment of functional activity in a cell-based assay or *in vitro* organ bath or tissue experiment. Biological evaluation will include construction of dose response relationships. Comparative activity relative to standard drugs is also commonly used as a control to validate the results in each and every assay.

Tertiary biological assessment usually involves a measure of *in vivo* activity. Drug administration is normally performed by the intended therapeutic route. An assessment of the likely duration of action of the test compound can be performed at this stage. The processes are designed to produce lead compounds for further evaluation and development. While development is continuing on one (or more) such compounds, the iterative process of discovery will usually continue until early proof-of-principle clinical studies have begun, in order to generate back-up candidates for development in the event that the original lead fails for toxicological or clinical reasons. The generation of these back-ups will depend on an assessment of the biological data as before, but usually with an added constraint of structural differentiation relative to the original lead. This is to guard against the back-up failing for similar reasons.

The project flow chart is important particularly for the parameters it uses to control compound testing. These parameters may vary during the course of the project; for instance the objectives may become more stringent once a lead candidate has been chosen, so that follow-up compounds need to be superior to the previously chosen lead. The parameters chosen should allow objective assessments to be made by the project team and facilitate decisions being taken on individual compounds.

The project flow chart acts to filter compounds, discarding them by increasingly demanding assays. Increasing numbers of compounds emanating from combinatorial chemistry programmes have necessitated the introduction of automated techniques for screening. The choice of protocol for the initial biochemical assessment is therefore crucial to the outcome of the project. Its correlation with functional activity both in cell-based and whole animal systems is important if the project is to be successful in finding valid lead compounds.

The techniques available to the biologist have greatly expanded through the possibilities of molecular biology. The advances in this area have been dependent to a large degree on automated techniques of DNA cloning and sequencing. Beyond simple sequencing, technology is now available for the determination of concentrations of every mRNA in a given cell, tissue or organism. It should become possible to measure such changes in response to stimuli, and understand mechanistic responses. These techniques as a whole are known as genomics. As an example of the kind of throughput now possible, Human Genome Sciences are now able to carry out 3000 to 5000 sequence determinations per day. The entire genome of *Staphylococcus aureus* was recently completed within a matter of weeks. Genomic information can identify proteins that are expressed on the outside of virus-infected cells or other organisms; this can lead to a new approach to vaccine production for a variety of diseases that are currently poorly treated, such as malaria and Lyme disease.

Molecular biological manipulation of pharmacological models has resulted in substantial changes in the outlook for *in vivo* pharmacology. Harvard University were able to produce strains of mice bearing a gene encoding a human cancer, and the so-called oncomouse can be used to test compounds for *in vivo* anti-cancer effects. Homologous recombination of embryonic stem cells allows the generation of predefined alterations of the mouse genome. One use of this technology is in the creation of 'knockout' models for which the causative gene has been removed. Mutations in the interleukin-2 receptor in man cause severe defects in T- and B-lymphocyte development; this is modelled in mice by producing strains which are deficient in the interleukin receptor. A similar approach has been employed to model Duchenne muscular dystrophy in mice.

Similarly, manipulation of biochemical models has been used extensively to produce genetically altered cells or biomolecules that can function in *in vitro* assays. This technology has been used extensively by investigators (e.g. at Allergan, now Ligand) searching for new, selective retinoids for dermatological diseases. Retinoids act through binding to certain transcription factors which lead to effects on cellular differentiation or proliferation. Rather than relying on whole human cell assays and looking physically for proliferative or anti-proliferative effects, molecular biological manipulation of the transcription factors, using reporter genes, has been employed to determine much more rapidly when the retinoid effect is produced. Scientists at Myco (now ChemGenics) have employed similar techniques to modify fungal organisms to produce bioassays which display different colours to indicate whether test compounds are selectively antifungal, toxic or inactive. These types of manipulation lead to biochemical screens which rapidly yield information on a compound's activity which can be read easily in a high-throughput assay. In this way, the process of drug discovery can be seen to be accelerated.

Molecular biology has opened the possibility of the therapeutic use of gene therapy. This approach employs active moieties based on oligonucleotides. As with the recombinant peptides and proteins mentioned earlier, the poor pharmaceutical properties of these molecules with respect to chemical stability and transfer across biological membranes has contributed to very poor oral bioavailability of these molecules and the problems in achieving significant advances in this area.

As a result of the potential evoked by recombinant proteins and oligonucleotides, drug delivery is increasingly a topic for widespread research in the pharmaceutical world. The achievement of good oral activity of these types of molecules by a means that does not abrogate the body's natural defence barriers against external toxins remains a significant unachieved goal of formulation technology. The need for medication to be administered by convenient routes and only once or twice a day has also brought controlled release technology ever more into the research frame. Novel formulation technology theoretically has much promise in these areas.[16]

It should be clear from the above that the traditional demarcation between chemist and biologist is becoming blurred by ancillary specialities such as molecular biology and by the involvement of computer technology as an enabling tool that has commonality to all disciplines.

1.2.4 Multidisciplinary assessment

It has been estimated that only around one in a thousand compounds that are screened is ever tested in man, and that the process of chemical design and synthesis is an inherently inefficient one.[17] The rest are eliminated as a result of failing to achieve the criteria required by a number of assessments stretching across multiple scientific disciplines.

The progress of a drug candidate through the very early stages of drug discovery depends critically on a weighted analysis based both on chemical and biological properties. In most cases, a biological assessment will predominate because the purpose of selection is generally to maximise activity and selectivity in animal biological models. In addition, the viability of a drug candidate will need to pay due reverence to the next hurdles it will face. Among these, toxicology, pharmacokinetics and pharmacodynamics, and pharmaceutical properties such as solubility and stability need to be considered. In fact, in some companies, the pharmaceutical properties of lead candidates may well be analysed before a single compound for progression is selected. Finally, although the large-scale chemical synthesis of any drug is usually a feasible proposition, the resources necessary, the time involved and the cost of raw materials are significant factors that should not be overlooked in choice of a compound.

All of these considerations need to be taken together for the greatest efficiency and probability of success for the subsequent development of the drug. This is conventionally done by committee, where each of the core disciplines is represented.

Beyond the research process, the research project needs to incorporate consideration of a wide variety of scientific disciplines, scientific, medical and commercial (see Table 1.1).

Some anticipation of these factors is advisable even before any practical laboratory work takes place, as well as during the discovery process and in lead selection for entry into development. The ability to balance the multitudinous factors in pharmaceutical research is one of the key requirements for success in this most difficult process.

1.3   PRECLINICAL DEVELOPMENT

The boundary between preclinical research and development is difficult to define rigorously and varies from project to project. One way of describing the transition into development is in terms of the way in which it is conducted, rather than what is actually done. In this sense, when a project enters a developmental phase the process becomes much more organised and determinative. The development phase normally applies to one or two development candidates, whereas research is conducted on many. Data are gathered in accordance with increasingly rigorous procedures, requiring adherence to good laboratory practice (GLP), or in the case of manufacturing, GMP, or clinical work, GCP. The uncertainty besetting research processes does not apply so strongly to development, while the economic implications and constraints of costs become increasingly important.[18] The involvement of a greater commitment, both in terms of resources and of finance, predicates a decision process which will have considered and planned a number of aspects of the proposed development. In addition to considerations of the compound itself, with criteria such as safety and efficacy, the strategic planning from an eventual marketing perspective is also often begun.[19] Compared to research, developmental activities can be planned sequentially, with time and budget lines more readily defined. As throughout pharmaceutical development, success of any individual stage cannot be predicted. However, a clearer vision of what needs to be done to arrive at the next stage is readily apparent. The work necessary to achieve that goal, and the time and money required, can be forecast.

A summary of the activities in preclinical development is shown in Table 1.2. Some of these activities will need to continue during the later clinical evaluation. Obviously this applies to chemical development, which will ultimately need to transfer to production scale manufacture. Pharmaceutics, such as stability, will also need to continue into the later stages. The more extensive toxicological studies

Table 1.1   *Requirements for assessment of research proposals*

CHEMICAL

- Feasibility of chemical synthesis
- Patentability
- Number of chiral centres
- Cost of synthesis

BIOLOGICAL

- Pharmacology; mechanism of action of the substance(s)
- Toxicological profile
- Bioavailability
- Duration of action
- Side-effect profile

PHARMACEUTICAL

Formulation

- Inactive ingredients: pharmacopœial status
- Physical and chemical properties
- Possible form(s) of application and reasons for its (their) selection
- Existence of polymorphs
- Patent situation
- Manufacturing process
- Storage conditions
- Dissolution behaviour

Production

- Manufacturing or acquisition of active substance(s)
- Capital investment required (or external sourcing)
- Production capacity
- Environmental issues
- Expected costs

MEDICAL

- Clinical trials required
- Indication(s); diseases to be treated
- Reasons for choosing the substance(s)
- Disease pathogenesis
- Standard therapy for disease (US, EU, Japan)
- Unmet medical needs
- Prevalence and incidence of disease

- Competitor activity in research and clinic
- Specialities and number of physicians attending the patients
- Disease awareness and diagnostic possibilities
- Superiority and/or shortcoming of the new product regarding effectiveness and tolerance/safety
- Mode, frequency and duration of application
- Compliance
- Dosage range per indication (compared to competing products)

MARKETING

General Aspects

- Strategic fit into the overall programme (e.g. synergy, competition, cannibalism)
- Image and competence of company in the indication

Demand and Competition

- Market volume, market growth, expected sales, expected sales growth
- Number and maturity of new drugs
- Competitors (importance and image in indication) (per country)
- Patient demography and behaviour
- Price level, price development, generics
- Therapy cost
- Therapeutic advantages and disadvantages

Marketing Overview

- Pricing and reimbursement status
- Registration requirements
- Cultural habits, medical schools
- Political, social, economic projections

Financial Analysis

- Cash flow
- Return on investment
- Net present value

Table 1.2   *Preclinical development activities*

Chemical development	Toxicology
• scale-up	• acute toxicology
• route investigation	• subacute toxicology
• process validation	• genetic toxicology
	• reproductive toxicology
	• teratology
Safety pharmacology	• carcinogenicity
	• chronic toxicology
Metabolism/pharmacokinetics	
• *in vitro*	**Pharmaceutics**
• *in vivo*	• solubility
• radiochemical synthesis	• stability
	• analytical methods
	• pre-formulation

such as teratology and carcinogenicity will usually begin prior to drug investigation in patients; however, carcinogenicity studies in rats typically have an in-phase duration of 2 years, and these will clearly extend well into Phase III of development.

During preclinical development, additional pharmacology will normally be conducted to define pharmacodynamics and detailed effects in a variety of *in vivo* models, to complement the work conducted in the research phase. In addition, effects in a number of other pharmacological models will also often be carried out to investigate other avenues of therapeutic utility.

Efficient handling of this phase of drug development is vital to a company. The costs of drug development and subsequent clinical trials limit the number of compounds coming through any particular development pipeline. Early positive data are crucial for the success of the drug candidate and have substantial implications for the financial well-being of the company, which depends on a strong cast of candidates passing through R&D. Compounds which fall outside the specifications set by these project management groups should be quickly, even ruthlessly, replaced by another new potential development compound.

1.3.1   Chemical development

The number of components in terms of people and of functional disciplines rapidly increases on passing from research into development. The complexity of the process also increases due to the immediate requirements of quantities of test material in the hundreds of grams or kilograms range. Hitherto, chemical synthesis has been conducted on gram quantities only.

In addition to the provision of larger quantities of material, the development of a robust process requires investigations of alternative synthetic routes. The eventual synthetic procedure that permits synthesis of large amounts of material may differ substantially from that originally used on a research scale. Alternative routes will also be required to be investigated in order to ensure secure patent protection for the development compound.

In the first place, the bench scale synthesis will need to be modified substantially or even abandoned in favour of a process that is practical on a large scale and amenable to the exigencies of a production facility. There are numerous aspects of a chemical reaction which may not permit extrapolation in scale. These include changes in surface area to volume ratio that influence heat transfer, the resultant changes in temperature gradient, mechanical differences in stirring (shear forces) and time differences in handling large versus small quantities. On a pilot plant scale, reactors are usually opaque, preventing visual observation that may have been of great assistance on a laboratory scale; chromatography, an almost universal research tool for compound purification, is rarely practical on plant scale because of the huge amounts of solvent needed.

Second, the process that is adopted requires analytical support to monitor product purity, reaction progression and the physical form of the product and to provide data on the impurity profile (such as identity of certain impurities) prior to use in toxicological or clinical studies.

Third, the process that is used needs to be validated and documented in accordance with the currently prevailing regulatory requirements. The latter will also involve consideration of environmental impact associated with the large-scale manufacture of the drug substance.

1.3.2 Development pharmacology

The transition into development for a new therapeutic agent depends on collective input and positive results from various pharmacological, pharmacokinetic, ADME,* toxicology and formulation studies. These pivotal studies shape the decision as to whether the lead compound has sufficient of the essential properties of a development candidate,

---

* Absorption, distribution, metabolism and excretion.

and at least some of the desirable properties which are imposed by the multidisciplinary development team which co-ordinates these studies. As far as pharmacology is concerned, great attention is paid to the possible side-effects of the drug candidate.

The recent trend in the US, and to a lesser extent in Europe, towards setting up new, non-traditional companies with highly focused medical research interests has involved much greater attention to research programmes that use biotechnology or molecular biology to define and understand pathophysiologically significant processes, and to build a therapeutic approach. These new companies are often fuelled by private finance or venture capital from investors and there is a compelling urgency for their limited sources of funds to be used only in activities which lead directly along a narrow preclinical and development path. The studies that take place in preclinical development are especially crucial for these companies that are much more exposed to financial vicissitudes. There are very strong reasons why compounds which pass through only a few primary, secondary and tertiary tests should be carefully examined for more than merely their efficacy in a number of disease models. Their safety profile in a wider sense is determinative for their value as therapeutic entities, and small companies are obliged to consider safety pharmacology studies before attempting to find a licensing partner.

In addition, in view of the pressures on healthcare costs, including prices, traditional pharmaceutical companies are adapting their development strategies and processes in the most cost-efficient manner, to bring drugs to the clinic faster and often with greater safety margins. Again safety pharmacology testing can provide information about a new therapeutic agent which defines whether it has an acceptable or unacceptable pharmacological and physiological profile in the major systems of the body, particularly *in vivo*. These tests should be carried out to GLP standard if they are to be used in the registration submission of the drug.

In many projects, a particular aspect of the eventual profile of the drug candidate may be considered sufficiently important for its evaluation to be made part of the research phase rather than being considered later in development.

For instance, in the discovery of ondansetron (Figure 1.3), the $5HT_3$ antagonist for cancer-treatment-induced emesis, the chemical candidates often incorporated an imidazole group.[20,21] The interference of this group with cytochrome p450 enzymes in the liver was known at the time (partly through Glaxo's sensitivity to the interaction of cimetidine with cytochrome p450, and the lack of this complication for ranitidine). As a result, the *in vivo* effect of drug candidates was

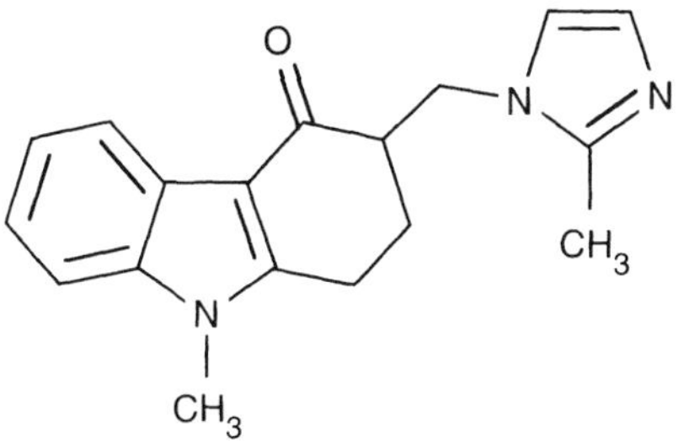

Figure 1.3   Ondansetron

measured on pentobarbital-sleeping time in rats early in the research process.

The discovery and development of ondansetron also illustrates another important aspect, that of choice of pharmacological models. Initial work on $5HT_3$ antagonists was based on their proposed therapeutic utility in a number of disorders, including anxiety, migraine, schizophrenia and cognition disorders. To date, no such utility has been proven in a clinical setting. It is ironic that the development of Glaxo's ondansetron as an anti-emetic conjunct to cancer therapy was based on reports of activity of competitor compounds from Sandoz[22] and Marion Merrell Dow[23] (now Hoechst Marion Roussel), whereas these companies have yet to be commercially active in this market. The irony is compounded, since the clinical use for which ondansetron is marketed, namely against cancer-treatment-induced emesis, was patented by Beecham, and Glaxo pay a royalty to SmithKline Beecham on the sales of ondansetron in recognition of this fact.

The ondansetron example points to the benefit of early examination of side-effects that were expected because of particular chemical structures made as drug candidates. Another example, from programmes investigating PDE4 inhibitors for asthma, relates to the mechanism-based side-effect of emesis. This undesirable property has been found for a number of chemically distinct PDE4 inhibitors both in animal models and in the clinic, with the result that most companies now in this field have deployed animal models of emesis early in the research process to eliminate compounds possessing this property.

These types of investigation would normally be considered as part of the safety pharmacological assessment conducted during the preclinical development phase. They have been moved to a research phase because of the likelihood of an adverse finding, which (as always) should be unveiled as early as possible. In all projects, the problems which can be foreseen ahead in development, whether related to the biological mode of action, to the chemical class and likely toxicology problems, or to the eventual therapeutic purpose and the position relative to competitors should all be considered as early as is practical.[3,19] Nevertheless, there are a number of safety tests which are conducted routinely as part of the lead up to introduction into human volunteers, and are rarely missed out of any conventional drug discovery programme.

1.3.2.1   *Recommended pharmacological tests*

The International Committee on Harmonisation (ICH) has worked towards reducing the differences in national regulatory requirements which could often be seen a few years ago in product licence submissions to countries such as the US and Japan as well as European states such as the UK.

The following tests, known as List A, would be required to provide a general and safety pharmacology profile of a new therapeutic agent in the major systems of the body (Table 1.3).

These tests themselves are described in general terms and there is an onus placed on the investigator to choose animals of an appropriate species, sex or age. Furthermore, there are caveats about the choice of the route of drug administration in some cases and this has to reflect the design of the clinical trial. The time-points at which drug effects are measured are also crucial and the doses or concentrations used in any test should reflect activity at expected subclinical and supraclinical doses. There is also scope within List A to examine predictable drug class effects in appropriate models to see what relative risk is inherent in a new compound.

Any unexpected positive effects, usually side-effects, can then be assessed by reference to the potency and duration of action of other known standard compounds for each test (e.g. sedatives or stimulants in CNS tests). A picture can be built up about these side-effects and at which doses they may occur relative to the planned therapeutic dose. This information might also have a bearing on other signs of toxicity seen in other systems at comparable doses. With all this information, a picture of the safety margins associated with a new compound is established.

If there are unexpected side-effects, then there is another series of tests advocated which breaks down the integrated test systems into simpler constituent organs or tissues, or may even allow the investigator to evaluate in another species whether this is a more widespread phenomenon than previously imagined. This is known as List B and is shown in Table 1.4.

Table 1.3 *List A requirements*

General behaviour
• multidimensional behavioural test—Irwin screen

Central nervous system (CNS) effects
• spontaneous locomotor activity
• general anaesthetic effects
• analgestic action
• anti-convulsant action
• pro-convulsant action
• normal body temperature

Autonomic nervous system and smooth muscle
• spontaneous contractions in isolated guinea-pig ileum
• effects on contractions to acetylcholine, histamine and barium chloride

Renal function

Digestive system

Cardiovascular and respiratory systems

Other appropriate pharmacological tests

With all this information available, pharmacologists can advise their colleagues in other disciplines whether the defined side-effect, which could even be offset by adjunct pharmacological therapy in some cases of severe medical need, compromises the safety and efficacy of the therapeutic's primary pharmacological locus. This is particularly important information for flagging potential problems in the toxicology studies—such warning can be invaluable in speeding development as well as in interpreting toxicological findings.

1.3.3 Preformulation and pharmaceutics

Development of the final marketed pharmaceutical entity has traditionally been the role of formulation scientists. The conventional solid and liquid formulations have been the bedrock on which medicines have been delivered to patients. Thus the formulation development group was only involved very late in the development process. This situation arose because there was no absolute need for formulation to be involved in the discovery and early development phases. Today the situation has changed dramatically. It is absolutely necessary for pharmaceutics specialist expertise very early in the process—drugs need to be designed with delivery components in

Table 1.4 *List B requirements*

CNS effects
- spontaneous EEG
- spinal reflex
- conditioned avoidance
- co-ordinated locomotor activity

Somatic nervous system
- neuromuscular junction
- muscular relaxation
- local anaesthetic

Autonomic nervous system and smooth muscle
- pupillary membrane and nictitating membrane
- isolated organs (e.g. blood vessels, trachea, uterus, vas deferens, heart)

Respiratory and cardiovascular system
- BP and heart rate changes (elicited by autonomic drugs, carotid artery occlusion, vagal stimulation, etc.)
- heart *in situ*
- isolated organs and tissues such as heart, atrium, papillary, muscle, vascular bed, etc.

Digestive system
- secretion of gastric juice, saliva, bile and pancreatic juices
- motility, *in vitro* of stomach and intestine
- motility of the gastrointestinal tract *in situ*
- gastroduodenal mucous membrane

Other effects
- blood coagulation system
- platelet aggregation
- haemolytic potential
- renal function

mind, and this is particularly the case for biotechnologically derived products (see section 5.2.3.3).

There are multiple factors which have driven the need for this change. The days of the medicinal chemist failing to consider in his initial design strategies the needs of the pharmacologist, toxicologist and clinician are long gone. Today with the introduction of the technologies of combinatorial chemistry and high-throughput screening (*in vitro*) there is likely to be no shortage of 'hits' and leads, but converting these into useful therapeutics will be a major challenge. Experience already tells us that though it may take a matter of weeks to months to discover exciting activity and high potency at a new molecular target *in vitro* it may not be practical to take the compound through its preclinical safety assessment, let alone market a new medicine.

Although it is vitally important that pharmaceutical expertise is introduced very early in the process, it also has to be recognised that the life-cycle of successfully marketed products needs to be extended through more innovative and sophisticated formulations. Such specialised technologies are frequently the province of small niche companies who provide the technology to large companies on a fee for service basis or for a royalty on sales of the formulated product. Typical companies are Elan and Alza (see section 5.2.3.3).

Alongside the synthetic chemical efforts, an evaluation of physico-chemical properties such as the solubility and impurity profile of the compound needs to be made early in its development life. Since different particle sizes may produce different bioavailability characteristics, and polymorphism may also give rise to variable results in pharmaceutics or clinical evaluation, these are critical aspects for early study. Of course, it is sometimes the case that polymorphism may give rise to scope for patents beyond that of the active molecule or its method of production. Such a result was observed with ranitidine, which suggests perhaps that in successful business there are no problems, just exciting new opportunities.

An early assessment of newly identified lead candidates by the pharmaceutics group has advantages for accelerating the drug development process. Selection of compounds for development must be made not only on the biological activity, but also on the compound's intrinsic chemical and pharmaceutical properties. Properties such as molecular weight, lipophilicity (log P), acidity/basicity (pKa), solubility and the number of hydrogen bond acceptors and donors should be considered. Pfizer have developed a scheme that they call the 'Rule of 5'. For each compound in the chemical library, it is noted whether the molecular weight is greater than 500, its log P greater than 5 and if there are greater than 5 hydrogen bond donor or 10 hydrogen bond acceptors. Poor oral absorption and cell penetration is more likely if these factors are exceeded and this is indicated on the Pfizer database. This is a drug hunting approach. Early recognition that one is dealing in practice with active compounds that are 'brick dust' or 'grease balls'* and which are therefore undevelopable as drugs saves an enormous amount of time, money and frustration.

This is an area of the development process which can be handled reasonably well in large companies, given that the expertise is within the organisation and that it is made available at the critical interface

---

* Referring to the propensity for compounds either to be insoluble, or to partition exclusively into organic rather than aqueous solutions. Some degree of water solubility is of course essential for drugs to be absorbed and carried round the body.

of discovery and development phases. The only problem facing these large companies is whether the pharmaceutics facilities are sufficiently modern to accommodate the highly regulated operations which were once the province of only the preclinical safety assessment facilities. It is now essential that the pharmaceutics laboratories are monitored and controlled for compliance and environmental quality. Pre-approval inspections by regulatory authorities are now very much part of the pharmaceutical development scene.

1.3.4   Clinical development

The next, clinical, stages of clinical development are increasingly complex and costly. They are divided into three stages:

- Phase I studies the safety, tolerability, pharmacokinetics and sometimes basic pharmacology of the drug given in single and repeated doses to human volunteers.
- Phase II examines pharmacological and therapeutic effects in patients, defines dose response relationships, the therapeutic range and margin of safety.
- In Phase III, large-scale trials aim to demonstrate efficacy, safety, and (increasingly) examine cost–benefit and pharmacoeconomic parameters of the drug treatment. These trials employ the final drug formulation intended for marketing and commercialisation.

The decision to develop a drug implies that the profile from research studies justifies the commitment to all of the above. Because this commitment is a substantial one in terms of resources and money, it needs to be taken seriously. The involvement of senior management in this process is advocated.[24] At the start of the preclinical development programme, it is vital to have defined the clinical target and the route of administration, and to have some idea of what clinical trials will be required, and where they will be conducted.

In order to facilitate efficient and rapid progress as the first developmental stage is contemplated, a substantially increased level of planning across disciplines is required.

1.4   PROJECT MANAGEMENT

In acknowledgement of the complex and manifold studies required during development, most pharmaceutical companies have incorporated interdisciplinary connections into their organisational arrangements. The extent to which this harmonises, or competes with, the traditional departmental organisation varies. Companies organised along disciplinary lines into well-delineated functions can become strong in their specialised areas of know-how, but tend also to build barriers to interdisciplinary co-operation. This can present conflicts which hinder the smooth interlinking of tasks which involve transfer of information and work from one department to another.

It can be argued that the knitting together of these various disciplines is the single defining characteristic of industrial pharmaceutical R&D, since most if not all of the other operations are performed in whole or in part in academia (research) or CROs (development). Project management creates value from diverse scientific findings, since without it these findings cannot be transformed into a commercial product.

The make-up of the project team is of great importance to the success of the project. Representatives from all the key disciplines should be incorporated. The team should define the project objectives, from a strategic and tactical point of view. As a project progresses through research, preclinical development and into the various stages of clinical development, the key disciplines may change and membership of the project team will correspondingly change. However, it is important to preserve a core of multidisciplinary personnel who will have had continuous exposure to the project throughout a number of stages.

The project leader should have a broad understanding of all the scientific data that will be generated during the project; along with an ability to judge the quality and relevance of the data in respect of regulatory requirements and in comparison to competitor products. The project leader must have sufficient management support to command respect and to ensure his/her suggestions are adequately responded to; and finally, given the involvement of project members with different (sometimes competing) line-management responsibilities, it is essential that the project leader is skilful in managing the project team and in dealing with any conflicting priorities that may arise.

The issue of a 'rolling' project team membership is important if an overly large and cumbersome number of participants is to be avoided. Large teams can be more difficult to mobilise, each member reflecting a relatively lesser degree of involvement with the project's achievements. The project team's meetings should become the conduit for interdisciplinary collaboration and co-operation outside the meetings themselves, rather than being seen as an opportunity for members to illuminate their progress in an individual light. The purpose of the team meetings is to make decisions for future activity: these decisions should be acted upon without referral to, or amendment by, line management of project team members.

Project management is becoming increasingly used as a tool for pharmaceutical projects. Its benefit in pharmaceutical development is clear because of the complexity of the process. Herzog,[25] in a series of articles, has laid out the principles of operation and advantages of project management in pharmaceuticals. The ingress of this technique into ever earlier stages of the research process has mixed blessings.

On the one hand, detractors of project management techniques for first-stage research would argue that each pharmaceutical project should be seen as unique. In development, many of the processes are common to a number of different projects. In research, such areas of overlap are less evident, and the benefit from such an approach less obvious to understand. Second, it is far more difficult to plan research processes reliably (since, by their nature, they must be more or less unknown at the start) than to progress a compound through development. Janssen is a strong advocate of an approach to research that lacks strict plans and goals: research, by its nature, is unpredictable. Few could argue that under his leadership, Janssen's company has been phenomenally successful in getting original molecules to market. Out of a total of around 70 000 synthesised compounds, 70 have been marketed, with 30 more still in development. This represents a success rate (1 marketed compound per 1000 synthesised) around ten times the industry average (1 per 10 000).

On the other hand, in the real world, the experience of past successes (and failures) in pharmaceutical research does make it possible to set milestones and goals at relatively early stages in a research project. These objectives may be primitive and wide in terms of timescale, but their value is crucial to the effectiveness of the research process, since they specify direction, common purpose and criteria by which success may be judged.

Placing the research phase in a planned context permits an assessment relative to time of the progress of the project. There have been occasions when research even in an industrial setting, set loose from temporal constraints, can drift. The purpose and value of the research is inevitably linked to time: a successful programme that delivers a product to the market years after a competitor is usually not a commercial proposition. A project that is years ahead of its next competitor is correspondingly much more valuable. The number of years that one may reach the market behind the leader in a particular therapeutic approach is declining as the acceptability of so-called 'me-too' products is waning. Williams and Malick[26] have proposed an

Table 1.5 Drug development data times and costs of Merck and Co

Testing phase	Duration (years)	Costs ($m)	Success rate (%)		
			Wenzel	Recombinant Capital	Grabowski
Preclinical	1.5–2	5	50	75	
Phase I					75
Phase II	ca 2.5[a]	20[a]	20[a]	50[a]	48
Phase III	ca 3	30	60–65	60	64
Total	7–7.5	55		19[b]	23[b]

[a] Data for Phases I and II combined.
[b] Including probabilities for success in NDA review.

amended version of the project flow chart to include a temporal dimension. This is aimed to suit the needs of both project planning and scientific evaluation. Clearly, a framework which places the project at hand in the context of competitors' projects with similar modes of action or therapeutic end-points, is essential in today's environment.

An analysis over seven years to 1991 of 74 projects at Merck and Co. emphasises the statistics of this company's experience with drug development (see Table 1.5).

These data from Wenzel[27] define the preclinical phase of drug development from the assignment of a development lead up to, but excluding, Phase I investigation (i.e. excluding research). Using this definition, it is apparent that the preclinical phase of development lasts 1.5 to 2 years. Alongside these data on duration of each phase are estimates of the probabilities of success at each phase; comparative data from Recombinant Capital, a consultancy firm in San Francisco,[28] and Grabowski[29] are included in this analysis.

More details of the analysis from Grabowski[29] are shown in Table 1.6. In this case, the preclinical phase includes all work up to entry into Phase I volunteer trials, and at 43 months is correspondingly longer than that estimated by Wenzel. If we can take the two above tables together, this would suggest that the research phase lasts around 19–25 months.

Another revealing paper on the statistics of drug discovery, its costs and distribution of resources by functional discipline, is to be found in an analysis of the UK industry from 1985.[30]

The large amount of effort required by chemists and biologists and the relatively poor predictability of the outcome of their efforts has contributed to the perception cited above, that project management has little place at this early stage of a project. However, the increasing

Table 1.6   *Expected costs per marketed NCE (in 1987 US million dollars)[a].
Reprinted from reference 29 with kind permission of Elsevier-NL, Sara
Burgerhartstraat, 1055 KV, Amsterdam*

Testing phase[b]	Uncapitalised expected cost	Mean phase length (months)	Capitalised expected cost[c]
Preclinical	65.5	42.6	155.6
Phase I	9.3	15.5	17.8
Phase II	12.9	24.3	21.4
Phase III	20.2	36.0	27.1
Long-term animal	5.3	33.6	8.2
Other animal	0.4	33.6	0.7
Total	113.6	141.6	230.8

[a] All costs were deflated using the GNP implicit price deflator. A 23% clinical approval success rate was utilised.
[b] The NDA review period was estimated to last 30.3 months. Animal testing was estimated to start 4.0 months into Phase II.
[c] Costs were capitalised at a 9% discount rate.

use of robotics and computerised data handling methods may indicate a desire on the part of some companies, such as Glaxo Wellcome,
to tame the hostile probabilistic elements of the research process
through application of the law of averages. This approach seems
diametrically opposed to the hitherto advocated 'rational' drug design
process revolving around molecular modelling techniques. Current
principles of drug design are refocusing on the complementarity of
the rational and the haphazard, returning to the long-held principle
that a mixture of luck and judgement is required for success (see
section 5.2.2). If drug research becomes increasingly performed by
routine methods with the aim of reducing the time and variability of
the research phase, the ability of the overall process to be planned
reliably from an earlier stage of research may become more possible.

2
The Advantages of Contracts and Collaborations

2.1 ECONOMICS

In his widely quoted work on the costs of pharmaceutical research and development, Grabowski[29] estimated the cost of bringing a new chemical entity to market to be $231m in 1987. (Another estimate of $360m has been proposed by the Pharmaceutical Research and Manufacturers Association,[31] and more recent research by Lehman Brothers suggests that in the past 10 years this cost has rocketed further to $597m at 1994 prices.[32]) This figure is based on actual costs of $114m and a capitalisation element realised from a compounded rate of interest of 9% that would have resulted from investment therefrom. When divided by phases, as was shown in Table 1.6, the preclinical phase bears the majority of the uncapitalised cost. This is due to the attrition of drugs throughout the development process, requiring that the preclinical phase needs to be repeated a number of times for each successful launch of a new chemical entity. Because of its occurrence earlier in development it also incurs an even greater proportion of the capitalised cost, calculated as the uncapitalised cost plus interest over the development time at the prevailing rate. One modification that should be considered in today's climate is the improvement in regulatory review periods. Grabowski assumed an NDA review period of 30.3 months. The median period at the FDA in 1994 was 17.5 months, and improved to 16 months during 1995.[33,34]

Recent analysis of the economics of pharmaceutical R&D points out the dilemma confronting the industry today when faced by increasing regulatory demands, concern about prescription costs (such concern even recently voiced by the veteran writer and protagonist for the pharmaceutical industry, Harry Schwartz[35]), in addition to decreased patent life and greater research and development costs. The industry's initial reaction has been to reduce further the outlay on R&D. Such expenditure is risky and no longer guarantees a return, the argument goes; but without such expenditure new drugs cannot result. Following the trend in downsizing of the past five years, industry pundits are now re-evaluating, recognising the central part to be played by R&D. Without it, the industry has no future. The report by Lehman Brothers[32] emphasises this point, and suggests that outsourcing of R&D will be the way forward. In order to be able to use the most up-to-date technology, large pharmaceutical companies will need to collaborate with specialists. The economic advantages of such a shift are suggested to be huge. The report produces figures suggesting a collaborative project is estimated to cost $40m to develop a product, whereas an in-house alternative costs $205m. The return on collaborative projects is 475%, versus 225% for in-house projects.

The quantitative accuracy of any of the above figures, which suggest widely varying costs of product generation, must be open to question. But the relative difference between in-house and collaborative costs is sufficiently large to require further investigation by large companies. One immediate reaction to these figures could be that they are based on inaccurate assumptions; after all, contract-based drug R&D, especially at the early stages of research, is much less well known than the traditional methods. The database of successful drug registrations by this means may be far too small to make any statistical analysis. It is only as a result of future experience that the economic advantages or otherwise of the collaborative approach can be better assessed. The reasons why contracts and collaborations might lead to a more cost-effective method of drug R&D are dealt with in subsequent sections of this chapter, but there is one concrete economic advantage that is worth mentioning now.

Slippage, or delay, is a common, almost universal term in project plans. There are legitimate reasons of ill-luck, and illegitimate reasons of poor planning that underpin this phenomenon. Estimates from Recombinant Capital show that the chances of delay, although low at each individual stage, mount up and add an extra year to the mean expected development time for a new drug (Table 2.1).

In-house projects suffer substantial costs from slippage. Not only is the immediate planned study put back, but there may well be consequential delays from a less efficient project plan. Moreover, the people whose time has been booked for the project have to be reallocated to something else, since they remain on the payroll (their costs are fixed). Contracted studies are subject to variable-cost

Table 2.1 *Chances of delay at each stage of development*

Stage	Time (years)	Chance of delay of:	
		1 year	2 years
Preclinical	2	10%	5%
Phase I	2	10%	5%
Phase II	2	10%	5%
Phase III	2	10%	5%
Mean expected time for development 9 years			

accounting. If the study is delayed six months, the cost remains the same.

This argument applies to one of the problems of delay, namely increased cost of development. There are at least two other problems with delays. First, delays lead to later arrival on the market, which in the case of competitor projects can lead to loss of market share. Second, delays in development eat into active patent life; costs are truly related to the loss of revenue at the end of the patent life of the product. W Leigh Thompson, retired Chief Scientific Officer of Lilly, has estimated that for a product with peak sales of $1bn a year, a delay of one day will erode at peak sales rates, and cost $2 737 851. This is a remarkable sum.

Finally, one of the arguments often used against using Contract Research Organisations (CROs) for developmental studies is that, per study, they are much more expensive. This may be because CROs spend a lot of time promoting their capabilities, that they occasionally underutilise their resources, and so on: they after all have their overheads to support and profits to return. However, a recent analysis of a series of clinical studies conducted by Hoechst Marion Roussel[36] suggests that this is not the case. First, the successful CRO must achieve an 80–85% proportion of total personnel hours as billable in order to maintain profitability. In comparison, sponsor companies are estimated to net around 70–75% of available staff hours for direct project work. Second, the average salaries and benefits for CRO personnel are generally lower than those of their sponsors; a similar comment applies to administration and facilities overheads. Set against these factors is the need for a CRO to return a profit, which is not an element that applies to calculations for in-house alternatives. In practice CROs are generally within 10–15% of the cost of in-house alternatives—sometimes cheaper, sometimes more expensive. If the trend towards use of outsourced work continues, the margin in favour of the CRO will improve; the CRO will

$$\text{\#NCE per year} = \frac{R_{1\text{-}n}}{C_{NCE} \cdot t}$$

$$C_{NCE} = C_{project}/P_r \cdot P_d$$

where:

$R_{1\text{-}n}$ = sum of R & D budgets for top n pharma companies
C_{NCE} = cost per NCE
$C_{project}$ = cost per project
t = turnover time of NCE research projects
P_r = probability of drug entering development
P_d = probability of drug entering market

Figure 2.1   *Relationship between R&D costs, risk, time and output of NCEs in pharmaceuticals*

be better able to utilise its resources effectively and efficiently, and they will need to spend less time and expense selling themselves with mass-mailed glossy brochures.

The arguments of expense applied to the outsourcing of studies to CROs certainly do not apply to work carried out in an academic environment. The funding for Zeneca's collaborative effort with the University of Cambridge on combinatorial chemistry which is worth £1.1m over five years from 1995 to the University to fund a cohort of 12 PhD students represents something of a bargain compared to Zeneca's costs for the same number of graduates employed in-house (see p. 137).

In summary, the economic argument for the use of contracts and collaborations in pharmaceutical R&D is simply that such arrangements can cut the cost of bringing a new drug to market. The actual reasons for this phenomenon are examined in more detail in the following sections (2.2 to 2.8). The equation shown in Figure 2.1 indicates that there are a number of variables that may be modified to decrease the cost per NCE. In addition there are additional arguments based on structural elements of drug discovery—how it is organised, how the scientists are motivated and how it can deal flexibly with the increasingly rapid changes in science—that may be brought to bear through collaborative arrangements.

2.2   EFFICIENCY

The efficiency argument for outsourcing says simply that costs can be reduced, because resources are better utilised for more than one client by such means. This is in part an argument for reducing developmental costs rather than research costs, but since these are a major component of bringing a product to market, their minimisation is essential. The argument as it applies to research is based on the fact that information and learning experiences are shared.

Pharmaceutical research is by its very nature secret. This factor has been behind the historical preference for the pharmaceutical industry to conduct all, or nearly all, of a new drug's research and development work in-house. Inevitably, this has led to repetition. This is particularly the case in therapeutic approaches that have at one time or another become very popular. It can be argued that such competition and repetition will at the same time lead to slightly different approaches of different merits. Such diversity can be seen as beneficial overall to healthcare as leading to greater choice for patients and physician. Out of, say, 20 competing products, only two or three will take the majority of the market. But there can be no doubt that there is redundancy, and very similar approaches are often taken towards the same goal. In order to maintain an edge on the competition, leaders in any particular field will be reluctant to reveal the totality of their approach. Different companies guard their technology with different degrees of propriety.

Each programme begins with either a little knowledge, or what little can be gleaned from publicly available information. A new entrant into a field will need to travel the same or a similar route to their competitors. Much effort is spent in cloning human biomolecules, perfecting enzyme and receptor assays, developing *in vivo* pharmacological models and understanding the relative merits or otherwise of a particular series of synthetic targets. In so far as the learning process is repeated many times, this is clearly an inefficient process.

An example of the potential benefits of pooling of resources is in *in vivo* pharmacology. Development of good, robust models of disease processes is time-consuming and dependent on nuances which are not easily grasped by the inexperienced. This may particularly be the case in transgenic animal models, such as are now being extensively investigated for a number of human diseases. Harvard University chose to patent its oncomouse, a breed of mouse that is destined to develop human cancer. As a result, many pharmaceutical companies have chosen to develop their own transgenic models, essentially replicating Harvard's discovery but not violating patent laws which generally do not apply for research purposes (see also section 5.2.3.2). Perhaps Harvard would have benefited more from offering a licence to a CRO, who could then have offered this model as a service, and repaid a royalty to the University. A contract research organisation in an industrial (or academic) setting can offer specialist services to a number of pharmaceutical companies. In so doing, specialist knowledge can be spread across a number of clients. One difficulty that has to be tackled is the separation of what may be called generic know-how from proprietary knowledge possessed by the CRO. However, such organisations regularly field such problems, and deal with them in the best way that maintains their reputation for integrity.

As will be dealt with in chapter 3, there are a number of difficulties in outsourcing discovery chemistry. Despite this, the new technology of combinatorial chemistry has been the terrain of a large number of alliances between small and large companies. The principle of increased efficiency and application of the most advanced technological know-how to a number of clients underpins this phenomenon. This subject is dealt with in more detail in section 5.2.1.2.

An example of the wider dissemination of technology even from within large pharmaceutical companies is evident from Parke Davis corporate research at Ann Arbor. This company has been in the forefront of the new wave of combinatorial chemistry. Part of their proprietary expertise lies in the solid phase work of Dr Sheila Hobbs DeWitt, and her Diversomer® technology. This is a technique for high-speed chemical synthesis that permits the simultaneous production of a range of about 50 similar compounds in milligram quantities. In a move to commercialise this technology and make it available to a wider audience, Parke Davis chose to form a separate company: Diversomer Technologies is free to sell the equipment and collaborate even with pharmaceutical competitors. This can be interpreted either as a far-sighted strategy or one that offers the most immediate return to the company balance sheet. Parke Davis presumably felt the opportunity for utilising the Diversomer® technology had possibilities beyond their corporate domain, and that making it available to others was the best incentive for Diversomer Technologies to maintain its technological lead. The disadvantages of making it available to competitors were outweighed by the advantages.

Parke Davis' attitude to collaborations even with major companies is unusual and perhaps enlightened, in areas other than combinatorial chemistry. They have also recently agreed to work with BASF on research into interleukin-1 converting enzyme (ICE) inhibitors, sharing research to date and equal rights to resulting technology and products. No doubt this strategy is based on sound commercial principles; perhaps both companies felt that as individual entities, they were weak in this field, but that together they represented a significant force. The thinking behind this move seems designed to maximise the outcome from limited resources, and allows collaboration between the two companies in one area of interest without obliging them beyond that area.

Rather than looking at this question on the basis of scientific discipline, it can be looked at by therapeutic speciality. As scientific endeavour enlarges our understanding and the techniques available to us, technical specialists in increasing numbers of specific areas are required for pharmaceutical research projects. Large pharmaceutical companies can no longer afford to specialise in all therapeutic areas; many of the multiple approaches that are currently being taken to combat a disease such as cancer, for example, are individually associated with specialist know-how. Monoclonal antibodies, tissue-targeted pro-drugs, gene therapy and drug delivery are examples that may individually be better provided by specialists who are familiar with these techniques and their application to other therapeutic areas than by one company that seeks to build up expertise for cancer alone. Medium and small enterprises are even more caught by the requirement for technical expertise, especially if they wish to grow beyond a core technology which is limiting their business perspectives or is becoming out of date. Collaborative efforts may offer a way into new areas with minimum outlay, and maximum return.

2.3   RISK AND UNCERTAINTY

Risk has been referred to in multiple ways in this book. It is inherent in the drug discovery process. It is the single greatest frustration to those within the industry and the facet most poorly understood by those without, yet at the same time it is the life blood of the industry's profitability. Investors do not like risk, except in so far as it enhances margins on blockbusters and enables substantial profits to be produced. One has only to look at the reaction of the stock markets to the news of a late-stage clinical failure on a company's share price. Curiously, by this reaction, one would have thought that the investment community had almost assumed success would have been achieved. Yet, on the other hand, the often exultant reaction to good news suggests that this, too, is unexpected.

2.3.1   Risk of clinical failure

Risk can be divided into two elements: probability of clinical success at each stage of the development process, and probability of success in a commercial sense. In addition, costs of development will increase if delays occur (see above), though the exposure to this element can be reduced if the delays incur few increments in fixed costs, through greater use of external resources.

There are two aspects to clinical success. First, one needs to choose the right project; and then one needs to choose the right drug candidate that fits this approach to develop.

Research into the probability of a drug entering Phase I trials ever reaching the market makes dismal reading. In his review of the impact of cost containment on the pharmaceutical industry, Professor Jürgen Drews analyses the multifarious pressures on the industry today.[37] At the heart of the debate is the need for the industry to continue to produce new drugs, and the increasing difficulty of so doing. A mathematical analysis of the problem is contained in the equation shown in Figure 2.1. The cost per NCE (c_{NCE}) can be represented by the nominal cost per project* divided by the product of the probabilities of the success of the project in entering development (p_r) and concluding development (p_d). Drews takes the cost per project as $20m, from which the cost per NCE (c_{NCE}) is $500m, where p_r and p_d are assumed to be 0.4 and 0.1 respectively.

A key conclusion of this analysis is that the world-wide pharmaceutical industry is currently producing too few drugs per year. One of the primary means of increasing the number of NCEs is to decrease the cost of each one, whereupon the available research spending may be better distributed, as shown by the equation above. Other obvious approaches are to adjust the variables p_r and p_d, which may perhaps be the result of improved drug discovery technology or improved drug discovery organisation. This analysis is based on a probability of success over Phases I to III (p_d) of 10%. Grabowski[29] concluded from a survey in 1987 that only 23% of drugs that enter Phase I are eventually approved by the FDA (Table 1.4). These probabilities were divided into 75% for entry into Phase I, 48% for Phase II and 64% for Phase III and NDA filing combined. The cost of failure was implicit in the headline figure of $231m for an NCE introduction in the 1980s. This figure and the enormous risk associated with clinical drug development have been factors of great concern to the biotechnology sector who are more exposed by virtue of their size to risk elements. These companies have sought to reduce the risk of failure. Recombinant Capital have analysed the commercial elements of biotechnology drug discovery. They conclude similar probabilities of attrition throughout the development process

---

* This figure is lower than the cost to take a drug throughout research and development, even assuming this process was certain, since it represents an aggregate cost of all projects, including those that are aborted long before they reach the NDA approval stage.

to those of Grabowski, but less pessimistic than those of Drews. Some companies, notably British Biotechnology, saw possibilities in 1990 for limited drug development (to obtain registration for Europe only) with a budget of £20m. No element for failure was included, on the basis that close scrutiny and good decision making can substantially reduce such costs. This emphasises the risk element, since this figure is estimated on an assumed certainty of clinical success. Certainly, to date British Biotech's track record is good, but none of their drugs has yet reached the market.

Reducing risk is one of the prime ways of maximising overall R&D effectiveness and reducing costs. Clearly, from Figure 2.1, an increase in p_d from 0.1 to 0.2 halves the cost per NCE. There have been many varied methods of analysing future financial prospects for a project based both on return if successful, and likelihood of success.[38] Predictions of value, for instance from the perspective of licensing, place greatly different values on the project depending on the method of calculation used; at the heart of the problem is the difficulty in assuming *any* return given the slim chances of reaching the market from the preclinical developmental stage.[39] One way to address this problem is to adopt a more global view, taking into account the overall outcome for a portfolio of products, integrated with time into a company's overall financial position.[40] Another way to view the commercial prospects of a pharmaceutical project during clinical evaluation is by analogy with the financial instrument of an option. As development proceeds, and the probability of a return increases, the value of the option increases in line with the expected return. If development is discontinued the value of the option is zero. This analysis imposes a commercial rigour on the decision-making process that guides the development of a drug. For all the scientific reasons that may underpin the continuation of a drug that has successfully negotiated, say, a combination of Phase II trials, if the commercial argument for a return beyond a successful Phase III is lacking, such progression should not take place. This seemingly evident analysis has some far-reaching consequences for research in general and collaborative arrangements in particular.[41] Because late-stage development is the most costly of all the stages in bringing new products to market, it is essential that the candidates for such treatment represent those most able to command a large return on investment. Indeed, the more choice available from successful early-stage development, the better the financial returns.

Rather than looking at the chances of success of a single drug candidate, the other aspect of clinical risk relates to an approach based on an assumption of the importance of a particular biochemical process in a certain disease. Most companies focus their research and development activities on projects in specific therapeutic areas. Some have integrated their research efforts world-wide, so that groups within the same company need to collaborate on a world-wide level. This in itself is a response to a previous era of burgeoning approaches to disease, but even so, no company can investigate all approaches to the diseases for which it has, or seeks, a commercial interest. The present situation is destined to become more complicated in the future.

The discoveries emanating from the human genome project promise to increase greatly the number of approaches to disease management.[42] The chromosomal locations and sequences of approximately 100 000 genes are currently being defined. It is difficult to foresee the amount of data that will eventually be produced from this project, but it is likely that within it will lie clues to something in the region of 3000 inherited diseases, produced as a result of mutations or abnormalities in single genes. In addition to traditional targets, such as enzymes and cell-surface receptors of subtypes hitherto unknown, there will be entirely new types of biological targets, such as transcription factors, signal/transduction proteins, intracellular receptors and regulatory proteins. Genomic sciences will unveil codes for secreted proteins that may become therapeutics in their own right (see section 5.2.3.1). Many of these targets may prove to be intracellular. There are already drugs such as the steroids which act on the cell nucleus, and others such as cyclosporin which act through inhibition of the action of NF-AT, rather than the extracellular receptor or enzyme typical of much other current therapy. The powerful long-term effects of such drugs, mediated through their impact on gene expression, suggest that transcription factors and 'nuclear receptors' may become increasingly popular targets for intervention in the future. A further aspect of the importance of genomics is evident in the potential for use in genetic diagnostic procedures. This field has applications in many areas, with moral and ethical considerations, such as use on the unborn child, and in assessment of life insurance premiums. Genetic diagnostics also has a number of potential applications in identification of patients at greatest risk, and in determining whether, and which, therapy is most likely to elicit the desired result. There is an increasing feeling that genetic profiling before prescribing a drug can offer greater success rates for certain kinds of drug treatment.

Opinion as to the usefulness of genomic information *per se* is divided: there is a great deal of difference between sequence information and functional information. An analogy from an earlier generation of biology was to be found in the field of serotonin research. Knowledge of this chemical as a mediator of smooth muscle contraction originated in the mid-nineteenth century but it was not until over a hundred years later that the material was isolated as a possible cause of high blood pressure. Serotonin has manifold effects on the central nervous system and on the peripheral vasculature and gut, leading to a confusion in the literature about its role that persisted up until the 1980s. The basis for the confusion lay in the diversity of receptors for serotonin (now numbering 15) and the different effects that activation of these receptors could produce in different parts of the body. Whether or not gene products in general turn out to be as complicated in their function as serotonin (or even more complicated) remains to be established, but understanding them with today's techniques is likely to be a quicker process. This may be possible from experiments involving genetic manipulation of mice to prevent expression of the biological molecule under consideration; such 'knock-out' species will become a useful tool for determination of gene function. Certainly there are examples at the other extreme, such as cystic fibrosis where the absence of a gene product has been unequivocally associated with a disease. Genomic science is unlikely to be separable from other sciences traditionally important for the discovery and development of new medicines, and needs to be integrated into the overall multidisciplinary environment for pharmaceutical research. Despite the controversy as to the eventual usefulness of this science, pharmaceutical companies do not feel they can ignore the tremendous advances that are being made, lest they are left behind by their competitors. There is tremendous potential for the identification of numerous starting points for many research projects. The approaches to these targets may involve gene therapy in addition to the classical small molecule methods of correcting a particular aberrant biochemical process.

It is likely that the work to identify and characterise a target may prove to be at least as difficult and time-consuming as that to identify a lead molecule and optimise it for developmental candidature. This posits a project structure in which much basic pharmacology will need to be carried out after gene sequence data are known, but before synthetic chemistry can start, whereas most pharmaceutical projects that are currently undertaken employ relatively little of this kind of preamble.

When viewed in this light, in order to provide the best opportunities for the discovery of the blockbuster drugs of the future, larger numbers of research approaches need to be investigated, and greater amounts of work will be necessary to validate them as having therapeutic potential. Some commentators go further, predicting that genomic research will revolutionise pharmaceutical discovery. Operating these projects through partnerships with academia and start-up companies offers the only realistic way for even a very large company to maintain its involvement with a large number of therapeutic approaches. Moreover, as regards lead identification, the availability of synthetic libraries derived by combinatorial technology places small companies in a much more competitive position than was the case historically, when large companies had a substantial advantage from access to substantial collections of compounds previously synthesised by in-house chemists, together with natural products.

The Lehman Brothers report[32] has estimated that small specialist companies will supply at least half the expertise for discovering and developing the next generation of new medicines in the first decade of the twenty-first century. In this way, large companies can broaden their fields of endeavour without establishing a long-term commitment that they may wish to change at a later date. They may retain an interest in more fundamental research than could be justified in-house, while at the same time small technology providers develop the deep, long-term experiences to allow them to best serve their partners.

There are a couple of reasons why outsourced discovery projects should be less risky than in-house ones. First, the view that can be taken of such projects by a sponsor is typically more dispassionate, leading to a more objective, better analysis of the best collaborative projects and lead candidates. Second, when the collaboration is with a small research project provider, the onus is upon that provider to minimise the risk to themselves of failure. Of course, a large company is subject to the same incentives, and is also likely to favour less risky in-house projects. However, for a small company, the incentive is stronger, it is in fact an imperative. In any large pharmaceutical company, there are examples of projects that were begun with poor prospects of success. Any small company risks its very existence in pursuing such projects. This is also reflected in the ability of the company to raise money from venture capitalists and the stock market. The process of raising funds, although not scientifically rigorous, nor of course guaranteeing a return, perhaps imposes a greater discipline and self-examination of the risks involved by the founders of the company, than does a proposal from within a pharmaceutical company.

There is a more cynical side to this subject. Collaborations often involve an unequal distribution of risk. Since it is generally recognised that the greatest risk is at the early stages of the project, research alliances or collaborations in which a small company conducts the research result in them taking a larger proportion of the risk. (Equally, such companies are least able to withstand the shock of failure.) By comparison, the exposure of the larger company is more tilted to developmental expenditures which it will not embark upon unless the risk element is satisfactory. From a purely financial point of view, the large pharmaceutical companies can gain access to high-quality research for a smaller sum, and at a risk premium, compared to projects generated in-house. This is not to decry the quality of the research carried out in larger companies, it is to point out that the large pharmaceutical company engaged in a search for a research partner can pick and choose the project of maximal probabilistic return, while at the same time absolving itself of the uncomfortable need to decide how and when to abandon in-house efforts. Large companies cannot remove themselves from risk entirely, but they can reduce it in its most troublesome manifestations. By exporting risk, the overall amount of risk is not greatly reduced; it is merely redistributed, and falls more heavily on the small entrepreneur or academic.

2.3.2   Risk of commercial failure

Even when drugs have satisfied the numerous clinical and regulatory hurdles, and do reach the market, commercial success is not assured. The fact is that nearly seven out of ten marketed new chemical entities do not recoup their original investment (Figure 2.2). This figure uses the net present valuation of a drug to establish its worth. This evaluation is based on applying a yearly discount rate for revenues that are yet to be received, and a yearly revenue rate for revenues that have already been received. Despite this poor statistic, the profitability of the pharmaceutical business is assured by the rewards of the rare blockbuster. Peak revenues for drugs at the present time have been analysed as having a distribution shown in Figure 2.3.[28] The returns from each class of drug can be obtained by multiplying the peak sales revenue by the probability of those sales being achieved. The uncertainty of predicting the commercial return on a drug during its development is a substantial element of the risk equation of pharmaceutical R&D.

Outsourced projects employing a small biotechnology company as a partner are likely to involve research on a project with a very definite commercial end-point. Naturally, the desire for presenting the project in the most favourable light when an alliance is sought will necessitate that the commercial outlook is bright. Therapeutic indications of cancer and inflammation are popular with such companies because the likelihood of large revenues is maximised. In addition,

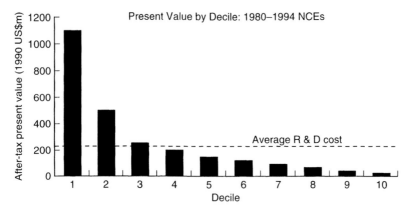

Figure 2.2   Most NCEs do not sell more than the average R&D cost. Reprinted from HG Grabowski and JM Vernon J. Health Economics. 10, 383–406, 1994 with kind permission of Elsevier Science – NL, Sara Burgerhartstraat, 1055 KV, Amsterdam

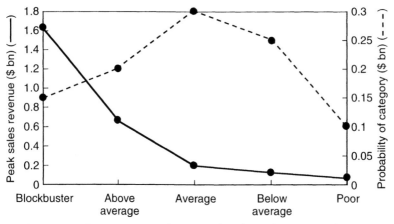

Figure 2.3   Categorisation of revenue by class of commercial return

the route through the clinic is smoothed by the primary targeting of acute therapy, since the clinical trial requirements are ameliorated. Chronic therapies are often considered as add-on indications.

Small research project providers will need to have done their groundwork to assure potential partners of the commercial merit of their offerings. Small market and 'me-too' opportunities are unlikely to be attractive for a sponsor company. Financial analysts of the biotechnology sector look at a company's rationale from a commercial perspective, which is likely to be more detailed than for an internal project. Finally, because of the greater ease of dropping out from research collaborations at greater risk of commercial failure, the proportion of collaborative ventures that deliver such outcomes (i.e. proceed all the way to market and then fail commercially) is likely to be less than the historic proportion, derived mostly from in-house projects (see also section 2.7).

2.4   FLEXIBILITY

2.4.1   Resource allocation

In a traditional, large pharmaceutical company, the resources available to project managers and research managers that enable pharmaceutical research and development to progress are defined by the budget set by senior company executives. However, in the allocation of such resources, managers are not presented with a blank sheet of paper. Rather, of the total budget allocation, up to 90% may be rigidly defined by fixed costs relating to existing staff, their fringe benefits, overheads (e.g. rent, equipment lease, heating), depreciation and allocated costs. The latter item covers company-wide service departments concerned with computers, information services, personnel, purchasing, engineering and the like. Additional technical support services such as animal handling, registration, data processing are also fixed in terms of cost. The portion of the budget that can be given over to flexible payments to cope with bottlenecks in a project is very small in comparison to the total spend.

This approach suffers in two respects. First, the ability to allocate resources to where they are most needed to progress critical projects is hampered. And second, such resources can often be left allocated to projects of lower priority. Thus the company is burdened with the expense of projects that do not offer the best chance of success, while being unable to devote sufficient resources to those projects that are most worthwhile.

The need to allocate substantial numbers of people temporarily from a particular discipline to a particular developmental phase of a project is a common problem for pharmaceutical R&D. Lack of capacity is the single most salient reason for the decision to contract out a study. It is widely recognised as an argument for outsourcing parts of clinical development, but it also applies, albeit to a lesser degree, during the preclinical stages of a project. A guideline as to the extent of outsourcing that is advisable is that one should be capable of using internal resources for the troughs of a project, and cater for the

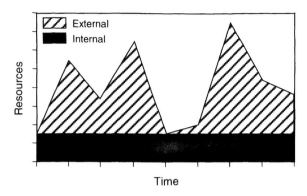

Figure 2.4   *Use of internal and external resources for variable project needs*

peaks externally (Figure 2.4). This is a favourite graph of management theorists, but one needs to ask how can one judge what is, in reality, the trough level of work required? Human nature, at the level of the departmental manager, is actually very unlikely to suggest that the department is overstaffed with regard to the trough level of demand, but certain to complain that the department is understaffed relative to the peak level of demand. In practical terms, the only reliable way to guarantee not to overstaff at the trough is to understaff for this eventuality and breed a strong culture of outsourcing, which in effect caters for some of the work all the time. There are, however, other reasons for contracting out from the point of view of human resources.

The impermanent nature of a pharmaceutical research project is fundamentally at odds with the long-term career sought by the scientist. This is compounded by the rapidly changing world of scientific endeavour, in which today's hot topic is tomorrow's bad news. Entrants into the pharmaceutical industry need to be versatile, since the nature of their work for the bulk of their career will be unlikely to be in the specific field for which they were hired. Indeed most large pharmaceutical companies take their obligations concerning such employees seriously and devote much time and effort to constructing exits from research for their maturing staff, to leave space for the younger entrants fresh from university. In so doing they seek to bring in new science, and take out the old. This is not to say that scientists are not able to keep up with developments in their field. Rather, it is to acknowledge that the frontiers of science to be applied in the discovery of the next generation of therapeutics are advancing increasingly rapidly. The skills now thought to be necessary for successful pharmaceutical research are fundamentally different from what they were five years ago. Although new skills can be taught or acquired, the fact is that the thinking processes change alongside the techniques. Older scientists will often approach a scientific problem quite differently from more recent entrants, filled with the most modern theories.

While this may be one reason for the increasing interest in contracting research, it does not solve the problem for those scientists left behind by change. Pharmacology is a case in point. Traditionally, pharmacologists tended to be categorised by their area of speciality, such as cardiovascular, central nervous system or respiratory. If the commitment to the particular speciality remains, year-on-year experience makes a scientist truly valuable in their specialist area. If the approach becomes obsolete, such as the use of histamine H_2 antagonists in gastric ulcers, the specific expertise attached to the discovery of such agents is no longer applicable. In this case, the reasons for the decline in the area have nothing to do with the science, but all to do with the lack of a commercially viable product in the face of generic competition from off-patent medicines. Pharmacologists expert in this area need to transfer their expertise to other areas of gastrointestinal therapy, or to other areas of pharmacology. Recent developments, particularly the increased importance of molecular biology in drug discovery, have made the pharmacologist's central position in drug discovery seem less secure.[43]

The challenges confronting chemistry are perhaps even more profound. A few years ago, the average chemist would profess to feel equally at home with a β-agonist as with a thromboxane antagonist. The therapy, the approach or even the types of molecules was of little import. Now, the advances are being made in automated techniques which work on solid phase supports, or in computerised techniques upon which 20 years of traditional medicinal chemistry expertise will hardly have touched. When such fundamental changes can occur so rapidly, with all the associated problems and costs associated with retraining and personnel changes, the long-term career prognosis for the highly trained and specialised scientists that drug discovery is based upon, is unpromising.

2.4.2 Accuracy and efficiency of selection

Aside from the difficulties highlighted above, there are traditional problems associated with recruitment which have not been resolved. The methods of the selection process hinge on a number of criteria, but despite the substantial effort that has been put towards them, there is little evidence that they are at all effective. A detailed study of these methods was made in 1988 by the then Institute of Manpower Studies (now Employment Studies), associated with Sussex University.[44] It concluded that the tripos of conventional methods employed by prospective employers, namely interviews, examination qualifications (curriculum vitae) and references, was little better than a statistical chance at providing the best candidate. For instance, from a group of three, the study concluded that the chances of the best candidate being chosen for a job were 35%, that is 2% better than chance. Although there are obvious problems associated with such selection procedures, the average employer was, at that time, loath to consider alternative methods of selection. Curiously, the research showed that one of these methods, psychometric profiling, was more effective than the usual techniques. Since this survey was conducted, alternatives to the tripos of conventional methods have continued to be developed, and it may be concluded that the advantages of techniques such as psychometric testing methods would be more likely today to outstrip the performance of the interview system. Certainly they are gaining in popularity as selection tools, but rarely is their evidence seen as more important than the interview.

The problem of selection is exacerbated by the reluctance of the employer to accept these objective analyses, partly justified by the difficulty of creating 'what-if' scenarios. Although the inaccuracy of selection is acknowledged, it is thought the best system available. Errors are difficult for an employer to acknowledge when they involve admission of a candidate into a lifelong career, with consequences for the company stretching out over decades. Selection procedures are also involved in promotions and transfers within the company, and again errors can and do occur, with long-term consequences. For all the downsizing and re-engineering currently in vogue, employers have great difficulty in applying objectivity to real individuals. This is not meant as a criticism, but it is nevertheless a reality that individuals exist in every company of a reasonable size whose careers owe more to the employer's concern for his employee than for his company.

Collaborative projects can allow access to the world's brightest and best. This is particularly the case with academic collaborations. The aptitude of the scientist concerned may not have been established in the mustiness of a sealed interview room. His/her personal qualities and ability to interrelate may not fit the profile of the personnel department's psychometric testing. But collaborations are judged according to record. Entry into them is determined by prior scientific achievement, and their continuation similarly dependent upon output. Partnerships in general are renewable only on the basis of satisfactory performance. The increased freedom of this relationship allows a degree of flexibility impossible in a world of lifetime careers. From the employer's perspective, the inefficiencies of selection are no longer a concern. Mistakes are rectifiable, and correct decisions validated by objective performance criteria. The market, as much as anything, will tell.

2.4.3 Access to facilities

The ability of many companies to conduct certain aspects of the research and development process is often limited by the physical requirements of space and/or equipment rather than people who can do the job. This may be so both for small companies, which may not have any capacity in certain areas, and for larger ones who find that the current facilities are overloaded.

Examples of this kind of need vary from, say, the requirement to do some toxicology in a specific animal species which is not handled routinely in the company's toxicology facilities, to the need to do some whole-body autoradiography, requiring specialised equipment, prior to entry into humans for the first time. Manufacturing equipment can be particularly costly and difficult to justify for small volumes. Contract manufacture, which is not strictly within the ambit of this book, is nevertheless commonplace by virtue of this rationale.

Naturally, if a piece of work needs to be done regularly, the argument for purchasing a specialised piece of equipment can be made on a costed basis. However, such costs should also include training, operator and overhead elements in addition to capital. It may actually be quite difficult to make such a justification if the need is predicated upon assumption of a project's continued success. Any decision to make an investment in a particular cause based upon such an assumption becomes an additional element of the exposure to risk should the project fail.

2.5 MOTIVATION AND ORGANISATIONAL STRUCTURE

Collaborative and contracted projects are by their nature impermanent. It is the impermanence that gives rise to the flexibility cited above. While on the one hand, perhaps this results in a feeling of insecurity, on the other it provides a great incentive for hard work and 'customer' satisfaction. The intensity of the incentive varies depending on the nature of the partner involved. CROs in general are highly motivated to do a professional job, to serve their clients well in order that they may return for some repeat business.

In addition to public sources of funding, an academic group may rely heavily on industrial funding to facilitate key research work. In the competitive world of science, such money serves to promote their impact on the scientific world at large. So-called 'soft money' may be used to fund research posts of a temporary kind (e.g. postdoctoral fellowships) but is now increasingly used to underpin even what are considered long-term positions. Clearly, when it is up to the lead researcher to bring in money not only for the group for salaries and for supplies, but also for his or her own salary, the incentives are intense. There is little doubt that such impermanency can place a lot of stress on the research group, which may be detrimental. The situation in UK universities has aroused much debate about the current ability to recruit quality researchers into the profession, particularly in certain areas of research.

For industrial CROs or for small companies that depend on alliances with larger companies, the commercial viability of the company depends upon obtaining and sustaining such contracts, and securing repeat business. In many ways this pressure is greater than that of an academic group because sources of public money are less evident. Although there are government grants available in the US and Europe for new entrepreneurial ventures, the award of such money is usually contingent upon submission of a feasible business proposition that is only partly dependent upon such grants. Within such ventures, there is a recognition that continued success is required for continued existence; that as they are small, individual effort is much more important than in a large multinational; and a certain proportion of companies of a similar ilk are likely to fail. Under these circumstances, and with the added financial incentive of stock options for continued success, dedicated hard work and a strong team spirit are widely prevalent. Motivation to succeed is little different from fear of failure.

This positive attitude should be compared with the sometimes bewildered atmosphere amidst the large multinational, which has recently suffered some form of downsizing, and turned the comfortable expectation of a job for life into dramatic uncertainty about whether a career beyond 50 years of age is possible. In this era of uncertainty, the willingness of a middle-aged, middle-ranking pharmaceutical manager to take risks is likely to be somewhat curtailed. One has to ask if the decision to abandon a project or to pursue a developmental candidate of uncertain prospects is likely to be influenced by considerations as to what is safer for a career, rather than better for the company.

The organisational structure of many large pharmaceutical companies is often designed to stress a unitary company image and purpose. Company hierarchy is deliberately aimed at the pursuit of a set of goals that are defined at the apex of that hierarchy. Large companies often have characteristics as a whole which reflect the personalities and desires of the most senior people in that organisation. While there are clearly reasons of efficiency that justify this order, scientists often feel their individuality is subordinate to the corporate ideal. Though the layperson's image of a scientist as a bewhiskered and bespectacled eccentric who spurns authority is rarely correct, creative talent is not optimally fostered in such a situation, even before the recent upsets amongst these organisations.

Small companies have much to offer a creative, capable and ambitious scientist. Their very flexibility referred to earlier does not give rise to an overbearing corporate culture. The lack of bureaucracy improves intellectual creativeness in general.[45] Scientists are recognised more as individuals than organisational fixtures. Since the success of a small company is more critically dependent on scientific progress, a scientist's work is valued more than their concordance to a company image. In recognition of this factor, there are pressures for large companies to unlock the hidden talent buried in their corporate structures. The advantages of flat organisational structure in small companies can clearly be used by large companies through partnering and outsourcing. The big challenge beyond that is to re-engineer the environment within the large multinational to maximise its creative potential. There is undoubtedly much native creativity buried in large organisations that needs to be revealed. Until the internal structures hindering bold ventures and forthright proposals within such large organisations can be swept away, the extent of the potential is not readily assessable, let alone realisable. To do so is of course intensely difficult, particularly if the advantages of large organisations with regard to co-ordination, efficiency and economies of scale are to be preserved, but the prize is huge, and there will no doubt be many attempts to reorganise internally in the near future.

2.6   SPEED

Speed is crucial for drug development. Although there will also be situations where the in-house alternative is more rapid (see section 3.6), the advantages of CROs in clinical trial management are becoming clearer as these organisations are becoming more experienced and better respected, particularly for large, multicentre trials. This is particularly the case for the large, multinational CROs, who have a global presence, and the capabilities to perform clinical work in Japan; access to large patient populations and extensive experience with investigator recruitment are other advantages that are attractive and useful for rapid completion of such studies. In addition, use of outsourced resources allows theoretically much more to be done in parallel during drug development than can ever be contemplated with in-house alternatives. Provided studies are not linked, or dependent on one another, the consequences for faster overall drug development using parallel project planning are well known.

As much as contracting allows an interest in a particular field to be rapidly curtailed, it also allows this interest to be developed very quickly. This is because the decision of the degree of involvement hinges on money rather than people. Hiring people, particularly good people, can take a lot of time. This is particularly the case when demand for such people outstrips supply. The time taken to recruit even temporary people when supply outstrips demand can on the other hand be surprisingly short.

An example of the benefit of external investigators may perhaps be found in studies that are designed to broaden the possible indications of a drug that was originally conceived for a single therapeutic purpose, but which was later seen as applicable for another. For a smaller company, the time to acquire expertise in a non-core area may be prohibitive, and there may be good reasons to consider external resources; for instance, there may be CNS applications open to drugs originally developed for peripheral pharmacological actions which require expertise not evident in-house. Studies such as these may theoretically be done well by an external biological investigator, and often from academia.

An example may be found in efforts to acquire an interest in a new area of technology, through investment with an experienced partner. A good example is that of Pfizer investing with Oxford Diversity, a subsidiary of Oxford Asymmetry, for the former's experience in combinatorial chemistry (see section 5.2.1.2). Glaxo's approach to this technology was somewhat different. In addition to its own in-house research, it embarked upon a collaboration with Affymax. Affymax was one of the first companies in this area, having been set up in 1989 by Dr Alex Zaffaroni, also a founder of Alza (see section 5.2.3.3). Glaxo's cognisance of Affymax's technological advantage led ultimately to an outright purchase of the company. The rationale for this event perhaps owes more to a strategic desire for predation than one for collaboration. Dr Brian Richardson, Director of Research at Sandoz between 1990 and 1993, has cited blocking of competition as one of the factors behind the formation of alliances with small biotechnology companies that are perceived as experts in their field.[46] Nevertheless, the Glaxo/Affymax story serves to illustrate one logical outcome of a strategic alliance, albeit one of the less flexible ones. As such technology becomes more commonplace, with several small companies in the US and Europe able to offer it, the price of Glaxo's acquisition may be seen as representative of the zenith of its value. Within most pharmaceutical companies, in-house research on combinatorial chemistry is taking place: thus, the use of external collaborations, while precedented, is normally used to supplement rather than replace internal resources.

In addition to the ability to buy into a particular expertise, collaborative arrangements of a large company with a small enterprise offer the opportunity of greater flexibility and ability to change with circumstances. It is generally agreed that small companies make and implement decisions faster than large ones. The responsiveness of small companies is probably related to their willingness to base their decisions on less formal processes, without the need for surveys or reports. Fewer people need to be involved in making decisions and delays of arranging large meetings are avoided. In certain cases, decisions can be made in small companies on hunches, and risk taking more readily accepted.

Time is a crucial element in drug research, as well as in development. Francis Bacon wrote in 1620: 'He that will not apply new remedies must expect new evils, for time is the greatest innovator.' Put another way, innovations that are behind the time are not innovations. Nor do they sell.

2.7 DISENGAGEMENT FROM UNSUCCESSFUL RESEARCH

As well as allowing a rapid involvement with an area, a contracted or collaborative involvement can be easily terminated if the business or research environment changes or research priorities are reconfigured. Termination can also occur for reasons of unsatisfactory performance. It has been stated earlier that scientific change is taking place increasingly rapidly, and hot areas of interest wane as much as wax. Disengagement can be even more rapid in the event of adverse findings. Such terminations can be swift and sometimes harsh justice on the weaker partner, but that is the nature of the world.

This is not always the case for internal projects in large companies, despite an increasing trend for analysis of projected returns on research projects. Such analysis is conventionally based upon probability of success, by phase; cost of individual components of development; and credible estimates of commercial value.[47] These techniques have long been used as pharmaceutical development proceeds towards progressively expensive studies. At later stages the chance of success can be gauged with greatest accuracy. But efforts to improve the efficiency of earlier stages of development, and even research, require probability assessments that are notoriously difficult to make. Objective analysis is tainted by subjectivity. Corporate psychology plays an important part here: in-house research projects are sometimes extremely difficult to curtail for several highly understandable reasons.

First, the project champion(s) is(are) often specialised scientists who have invested a good deal of personal energy in their field of specialisation. They are real people, known and often respected to the decision makers within their corporate body. Their belief in the value of their work may perfuse their estimates of success with a rose-tinted aura. Their influence is by definition greater when their exposure is greater, as is the case with in-house research. Even when the decision has been taken by senior management to curtail a project, the impetus to continue regardless from the lower echelons is strongly apparent (see also section 3.9).

Second, the human consequences of abandonment are much more evident and as a result hard decisions that much more difficult to make. One of the hardest reasons for research personnel to accept for abandoning a project is if competitor activity has made the commercial objective unachievable, while the scientific progress of the inbred project has continued steadily and undaunted.

Third, research and development directors are often loath to disengage from projects even when the objective chances of success are small in the extreme. Subjective desire clouds objective reality; psychology steers us away from the ignominy of defeat. Rather than risk the certainty of opprobrium of one's colleagues, one chooses the near certainty of pursuing a pointless project in the hope that the inevitable can be delayed—or even avoided entirely. It is strange but true that censure rather than praise often accrues to those who curtail unsuccessful projects. Their failure is to have allowed the expenditure of so much on a project that has not yielded a return, but their success in avoiding further waste is ignored.

Another way of looking at this is by extension of Drews' analysis described earlier (Figure 2.1). Research and development project costs increase dramatically in later development. Figures produced earlier (Table 1.4) can be graphically represented as shown in Figure 2.5. The most substantial costs are incurred in later development, and

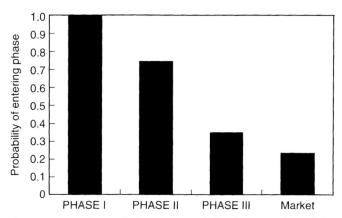

Figure 2.5 *Attrition of pharmaceutical developmental candidates*

anything that can reduce the fall-out in later development will be welcomed.

Without assuming that anything is done to reduce the cost of studies actually done, the overall cost of the programme can be reduced by steepening the rate of decline of the probability curve in early development. This was mentioned earlier as the 'fast-fail' method, to conduct the critical studies as early as possible.[3] Subject to the caveat that the end probability should not change, outsourcing may help to steepen the rate of attrition, by establishing an objectivity in analysis that is less evident in internal projects. By considering these pivotal studies earlier, even if they are not critical for eventual registration, success in them reinforces the confidence in the programme and may permit a greater number of future studies to be conducted concurrently, thereby limiting overall development time. Disengagement from a programme which is heading for expensive studies in later development is likely to be an attractive option for a sponsor unless it believes the work to date is solid and predictive of a near-certain commercial success.

These points are tremendously important to the advantages of outsourcing: external projects are judged with an objectivity, almost a cruelty that is just not possible with in-house projects. Perhaps one is able to harness the 'not-invented-here' (NIH) attitude to some advantage. Conversely, one only needs to consider the number of perfectly good compounds that are progressed to Phase III with no clear therapeutic market in mind to understand the human failings of R&D.

For example, Schering is one of the few companies to have developed a drug based on mimicry of a prostaglandin to have reached therapeutic use. Iloprost is an analogue of prostacyclin: improved hydrolytic stability was achieved through replacement of the latter's enol ether by a methylene group, and improved activity by incorporation of additional lipophilic methylene and acetylenic groups. The pharmacological effects originally noted for prostacyclin mimics included thrombolytic effects, cytoprotection for gastric ulcers and vasodilatation. However, the therapeutic gold mine awaiting the successful discovery of iloprost turned out to be (metaphorically) iron pyrites for Schering, who were able to produce clinical efficacy only for peripheral arterial occlusive disease (PAOD), a pernicious wasting condition involving loss of blood supply to the extremities which leads to ulceration and ultimately the requirement for amputation. Although iloprost inhibits platelet aggregation and causes vasodilatation, its activity in this disease was attributed through some elegant pharmacology to its ability to increase nutritive blood flow rather than total blood flow. PAOD remains a small market, and although the benefit attributable through iloprost to those small number of patients who have benefited is profound, it has not been a commercial proposition. The full calamity of the prostaglandin research afflicted many more companies than just Schering; in fact, Schering benefited a little (and iloprost is testament to their scientists' good work) whereas many others drew nothing from years of fruitless research. This saga indicates how initial objectives can become shifted by the persuasive arguments of in-house scientists; such avenues are not open to external collaborators, whose suggestions of alternative therapeutic targets are likely to be treated with substantial scepticism.

Another example where the original promise has not been fulfilled is British Biotech's PAF antagonist, lexipafant. Initially researched for the therapy of asthma, and perhaps other inflammatory diseases, the project was continued beyond the time when it was apparent that this therapeutic target was not achievable, because clinical trials of PAF antagonists were unsuccessful.[48] In search of a useful purpose for this drug, the company first chose sepsis, and then turned to pancreatitis, a therapeutic indication of little commercial value but which offered some chance of offering a degree of commercial return. In 1992 Glaxo took out a licence for this compound for oral treatment of asthma, and subsequent clinical evidence with newer PAF antagonists suggested that they may be more useful than at first thought. However, in 1996, after Phase II evaluation, the asthma trials were discontinued. There remains a chance of clinical success for lexipafant, in acute pancreatitis, and indeed Phase III trials are continuing. The commercial outcome will probably not be known for some years, but common sense indicates that the current prospects would not have accorded the project a great deal of enthusiasm if they had been known at the time the research proposal was originally made. The current strategy of new and frequently changing indications seems borne of desperation rather than obvious merit, and may indeed only add to the losses that can be ascribed to this research venture. Lexipafant is unlikely to bring in substantial funds if its indication is limited to acute pancreatitis, despite the fact that there is currently no approved drug for this indication in the US or Europe.

Failure to curtail a project at the most opportune moment can be very costly. Human factors, such as outlined above, can extend the unproductive use of research resources on a project that is unlikely to have a commercial return. At the same time, alternative avenues of research are not pursued because of lack of resources.

The financial position relating to a project is often not completely clear. It is rare for complete costings to be performed that include *all* the relevant expenditures, and which this author maintains should especially include lost opportunity costs. It should be borne in mind that one substantial, but hardly ever calculated, cost of failed research is that due to the failure to benefit from other (profitable) opportunities. Lost opportunities may not only be lost to an individual company, but also picked up by more successful competitors. As emphasised above, research projects can only realistically be undertaken within a narrow time window; once the approach has become commonplace, the opportunity for new entrants is limited.

By packaging a defined portion of the costs of a project into payments made to an external body, the assessment of financial commitment is made crystal clear. Budgets can be more easily set in advance, on a project-by-project basis, whereas the resources allocated from internal sources can often become less well controlled.

Glaxo's decision to modify its relationship with Amylin is a good example of a situation where collaborations can break down. The reasons for this move have everything to do with lack of scientific progress and very little to do with the realignment of strategic goals associated with the takeover of Wellcome. A moral lies behind this story, namely the risk associated with the raised expectations of the biotechnology industry. Glaxo may easily write this experience off to a false trail of ·pharmaceutical research, one that they like others have been down many times in the past, but Amylin has been greatly damaged by the failure, which goes to the root of its very existence. The original scientific theory was that raised levels of the protein amylin in metabolic disorders, particularly type II diabetes, suggested a therapeutic role for amylin blockers. However, as a result of more detailed observations it has now been discovered that late stage type II diabetics actually have low levels of amylin, perhaps again invoking the strange ability of the human body to compensate for imbalance. As a result of the development, amylin blockers are now being investigated in Syndrome X, which is associated with a cluster of metabolic disorders including insulin resistance, hypertension, dyslipidaemia and obesity. This shift has had substantial implications for the eventual commercial profitability of Amylin's research, and these implications are negative. The company's misfortunes were compounded more recently by the decision of their Chief Executive Officer, Dr Tim Rink, to leave to establish Aurora Biosciences. Nevertheless, having lost their attraction to Glaxo, Amylin have been able to recover through forging an alliance with Johnson and Johnson at the end of 1995. Their ability to raise about $30m in a further round of financing in September 1995 proved that it is still much too early to write off their approach and viability.

Similarly, Sugen had a collaboration with Amgen to identify novel signal transduction targets for therapeutic intervention in the fields of haematopoiesis and neurobiology from 1992 to 1996. The arrangement was terminated in January 1996 for reasons related to changes in 'research priorities', but despite a final payment of $2.5m from Amgen, the financial health of Sugen was not improved by the decision. Sugen was forced to immediately review its internal research programmes and external collaborations. The outcome of these deliberations has, perhaps unsurprisingly, not been the subject of a public announcement. Sugen has recovered from this setback, and has research collaborations with Zeneca and Asta Medica, but the loss of a major collaboration is a blow that small companies must be able to withstand if they are to survive.

These examples highlight advantages as well as disadvantages of collaborations. While the contractor such as Amylin or Sugen may feel overexposed to the impatience of their major partner, the system allows responsiveness to commercial pressures in a way that was not possible with in-house efforts. Of course the argument may be made that the commercial pressures are from a short-sighted investment community, that stock markets cannot foresee the value of long-term research. However, this is the imperfect system we must live with. A better one does not exist at the moment.

2.8   THE MINOR COLLABORATOR'S PERSPECTIVE

The above sections have concentrated on the reasons why it may be advantageous for a large pharmaceutical company to collaborate with external groups or companies in conducting some of their preclinical research and development. For CROs the service to pharmaceutical R&D is the mainstay of their existence. For universities, the access to industrial funds enables work to be done that could not be considered in its absence; the contact also provides evidence to government funding bodies of the practicality of their research, and attests to its quality. As a result, public funds are easier to come by. These points will be dealt with in more detail in chapters 4 and 5.

There are many advantages too for the small biotechnology company; in fact there is in most cases little alternative. Naturally, foremost amongst these advantages is the monetary contribution that accompanies such a venture. For many of the small emerging bio-technology companies their very existence as minnows in an ocean of sharks depends upon alliances. The cost of bringing a product to market in the absence of a larger partner is usually prohibitive. Even where it is financially possible, their experience in successful drug development is light, and the risk to the company should the trials fail make the go-it-alone approach unattractive. There are a number of salient examples where late stage failure has caused almost irreparable damage to the company. Synergen decided to proceed with its IL-1 receptor antibody Antril to a Phase III trial in sepsis but found the product was not able to reduce mortality significantly and was judged to lack sufficient efficacy to proceed further. As a result, Synergen lost a significant percentage of its staff through redundancy, and was eventually purchased by Amgen. A similar disaster overtook Centocor in 1991, following first its failure to effect registration through the FDA with the sepsis drug Centoxin, and subsequently by news of the clinical results that the drug caused 'excess mortality'. Centocor laid off 700 (45%) of its employees in 1992 after these events, and there were serious consequences for the biotechnology sector as a whole, which suffered tumbling stock prices.

Even when buffered through partnership, commercial consequences can be severe. Cantab were collaboratively developing an antibody treatment for kidney rejection together with Baxter when the product suffered a setback in a Phase II trial. Baxter withdrew its support, Cantab discontinued the product and substantial redundancies ensued although the company survives and has rebounded from this event, partly through establishing other collaborative ventures, notably with Pfizer for an animal vaccine. However, the advantages of the use of contract resources are shown by the example of Biogen, which used a series of contract research organisations for the devel-opment of Hirulog, and experienced no lay-offs when the drug was discontinued in 1994.

Establishing partnerships enables a small company to grow more rapidly than by developing its own products to the market. An example of this phenomenon is Oxford Molecular, which is engaged in products for computer-aided molecular design. This business is ancillary to the drug discovery process, and therefore does not suffer from some of the risk elements which make the latter so difficult. Nevertheless, the industry relies on software tools of this kind to facilitate the design of drug targets for synthesis. The business has been dominated by a small number of large players, but there have recently been some new entrants into the field, assisted by the rapid growth in the market for chemical software. Oxford Molecular grew at an astonishing pace in the early 1990s, and has placed particular emphasis on its contract design business. In 1995, the company announced a tie-up with Glaxo Wellcome under which the smaller company retained rights to the products it develops, while Glaxo Wellcome is able to develop the software further for its own purposes. In a further move into drug discovery it has formed an alliance with Yamanouchi to identify small molecules which are active against ion channels. Much of the work will take place at Oxford University; Oxford Molecular, like Oxford Asymmetry and Oxford Diversity (q.v.) draws upon its ties with the University for certain requirements and facilities, and this arrangement is an interesting model for University/Industry cohabitation.

Small companies who choose to become experts in a particular technology can form their own corporate culture in pursuit of this goal. For instance, they may require personnel of disciplines external to the core of sciences found in a traditional pharmaceutical company. These days, robotics is a key component of automated methods in discovery; the people who know about robotics are generally computer software experts, fluid mechanics, or electrical engineers. Small companies will be inclined to appoint experts in these areas with graduate or postgraduate qualifications; larger pharmaceutical companies often prefer to shift personnel from other areas and retrain. In fast-changing sciences, the former approach has much to recommend it.

Small companies suffer more extremely from the exigencies of time. Demonstrable success is a key ingredient to their attractiveness both to venture capital and to partnership opportunities. In considering a stock market flotation, the attraction to investors is rubber-stamped by the prior approval of a larger company, in the form of a collaboration of some kind. However, at the same time that money is being attracted in, it is rapidly being used up in funding research, and establishing the technology upon which the future is based.

The so-called 'burn rate' defines the success or failure of a company as much as its assets in the form of technological know-how or products. The mean annual burn rate of a group of 100 biopharmaceutical companies in 1994 was $18.8m.[28] This figure had increased from $6m in 1992, partly reflective of growth in the companies themselves. Small companies that regularly need to borrow tranches of money may therefore see advantage in contracting out certain non-core activities if this permits early arrival at a key stage, related to their ability to sell their technology or products.

The burn rate imposes a discipline, perhaps also felt as fear, which is tremendously motivating. Carl Djerassi's description of the total synthesis of progesterone, or the story of the Nobel prize-winning discovery of thyrotropin releasing factor (by Andrew Schally and Roger Guillemin),[49] are vivid depictions of the race to an academic discovery between two or more competitors. While these stories represent unusually strong ambitions in the minds of some highly motivated scientists, their motivation came from little, if any, concern about commercial reward. In today's climate of pharmaceutical research, commercial factors are part and parcel of an increasingly competitive and time-limited environment. Small companies who aim to ape the multidisciplinary character of the traditional large company in preclinical drug R&D are well advised to use contract research organisations or university institutions to fill in the gaps in their knowledge, rather than attempt to do it all themselves.

3
The Disadvantages of Contracts and Collaborations

Much has been made in the preceding chapter of the increased flexibility and ability to adopt new technology quickly through external sourcing. This is in reality a simplification, but one that is becoming common currency in the pharmaceutical industry. Management consultants blithely point out that other industries have been this way before, and that there is no *a priori* reason why drug discovery and development should not more closely model the car industry, where outsourcing is the norm. There is, however, a great deal of difference between the theory and the practice. Collaborative extramural work is more difficult than intramural, and as has been emphasised, intramural drug discovery and development is difficult enough. In the first place, there has to be someone offering the required service.

3.1 FINDING THE RIGHT PARTNER

Although it is true that partners may divorce as well as marry, one should not enter into arrangements lightly. An unsuccessful partnership will have cost more than money: it will have lost crucial time and opportunities that could have been fruitfully engaged in elsewhere. The choice of partner is not easy.[50] The numbers and variety of services offered by CROs and small emerging companies as well as in academia have increased enormously, and there are now around 800 CROs world-wide. Unlike human arrangements, one usually does not have the opportunity to affiance: one is committed to some extent from the start. On the other hand, one may be able to

Table 3.1 Factors to be considered by each side in research collaborations

Seller	Buyer
Money	Cost
Long-term commitment	Competence
Adequate internal resources devoted by buyer	Financial stability
Marketing presence of buyer in therapeutic area of interest	Quality

draw on past experiences, perhaps even make use of references. There is an increasing trend for companies to make more use of CROs and engage in preferred-provider strategies to enable growth in relationships from one project to another.[51] Some of the factors that are important from the point of view of each side are shown in Table 3.1.

The ambitions and goals of each party are often guided heavily by financial considerations. This applies particularly in the case of small companies that are hungry for both the cash and the prestige of announcing a collaborative venture. Negotiations on price can form the central element in large collaborative deals, particularly of the kind that involve strategic alliances. The risk factor that makes determination of the commercial worth of any deal is viewed from fundamentally different perspectives. One approach to reaching a compromise in any discussions is to share the figures underlying the calculation of the financial settlement. Although the financial element is crucial in all forms of collaboration, it should not be rated too highly. Table 3.1 indicates some of the other important factors. Long-term commitment is particularly important to the service provider; an over-jumpy attitude to adverse scientific findings makes successful collaboration, especially in research, very difficult. Reaching the right deal can have important implications for the future of both partners. Damage can be done to both by hasty decisions; a bad deal may be worse than none at all.[50]

On the issue of financial stability, it is currently rare for this to be an issue for consideration by the service provider, largely because the buyer in such partnerships is usually on a sound financial footing. Nevertheless, mergers and other changes in strategy can put the long-term commitment of the buyer in jeopardy, and the outlook for such changes should perhaps be a greater consideration for the service provider. From the point of view of the buyer, it is unfortunately not unknown for small contract research organisations to be closed for financial reasons, in which case either an entire study, or comparability between past and future results, can be lost (see section 3.10).

It is not straightforward to find specialist collaborators in particular areas of research. Although CROs routinely offer a range of common core services that are required for generic drug development, at the present time few CROs offer drug discovery services (and none offer basic research). Although a number of preclinical development services are provided, such as safety pharmacology, pharmaceutical sciences and toxicology, there are few bespoke services. Finding the right partner for research work from the traditional CRO field is not easy, given the specialisation that is inherent in the particular drug research project at hand, and the choice is not wide. In this regard, the key ingredient is information. There is no single source of detailed information of this kind, although Technomark publishes separate directories of CROs for both Europe and North America,[52] and a useful collection of non-clinical research and consultancy services is contained within the Soteros Directory.[53] Oakland consultancy publish a list of academic contacts relating to Chemistry and Biosciences.[54] Another growing source of information is the World Wide Web. Current sites of relevance and increasing value are represented at http://www.catosource.com, http://www.recap.com and http://www.biospace.com. However, much of the key information required for evaluation of opportunities in the academic sphere, and in basic science in general, comes from personal knowledge and contacts, and from keen observation of the scientific literature. Awareness of the possible partners for a particular piece of work, as well as for the rationale of the work in the first place, requires much broad knowledge. This knowledge needs to be complemented by effective systems of information gathering and reporting (see section 6.4).

Universities are often a better source for specialist investigators, and are often good for research collaborations, but matching academic aims with those of the pharmaceutical industry is not straightforward (see section 3.5 and chapter 4). Now that long-distance communication is easier than a few years ago, the possibilities for the correct partner can be found world-wide. However, the very breadth of the search domain makes the choice more difficult.

3.2 COST

The arguments for the improvements in economics of pharmaceutical R&D have been made in chapter 2 as though they were only on one side. In fact, the amount of money that changes hands in some of the more celebrated alliances that have been formed in recent times between the biotechnology sector and their large pharmaceutical partners would suggest that economic advantages may be hard to come by. The average pre-commercial payment that is extracted from large companies is increasing as this method of conducting research becomes more widespread, and as some of the small companies involved find the demand for their services permits such inflation. The principles behind the commercial agreement that is ultimately reached can be said to include those of supply and demand, and the more mature providers that are relatively flush with funds can afford to wait for the partner that is willing to pay their price. Even though the figures that reach the headlines for the value of alliances are heavily inflated by the inclusion of contingent amounts (e.g. milestone payments and royalties on a hypothetically marketed product), political alliance payments from large pharmaceutical companies to the biotechnology sector in 1995 totalled $3.6bn.

Detractors of the partnership argument may well point to the illogic of the disbursement of substantial funds from an industry that remains inherently profitable (i.e. large pharma) into the hands of the venture capitalists. Surely, there must be a better way of handling the situation; after all, the wisdom of the senior executives with many years of experience in this high technology industry cannot reasonably be surpassed by young, relatively inexperienced and scientifically poorly literate financial analysts, and by a crowd of investors who are unfamiliar with the difference between sound science and hype.

This argument strikes a certain resonance with the realisation that some of the stock prices of companies in the biotechnology sector are based on expectations of future profits that may be difficult, if not impossible, to achieve. However, it is important not to extrapolate this argument across the outsourcing industry as a whole. The advantages of outsourcing remain as set out in the previous chapter. The ways of achieving the advantages rely on the suitable choice of partner, and the problems that may afflict the biotechnology start-up company are certainly not the same as those that affect the CRO industry or academia. CROs are not subject to the same financing regimen, nor are they likely to be as avaricious in their charges for the alliances that they form (since the competition is intense). Some companies are also more at home with partnerships based on straight contracts with CROs because they are less cumbersome to operate, and allow greater flexibility in choice of partner for different stages and different components of the pharmaceutical R&D process. On the other hand, a partnership with a CRO does not imply the same input of invention (in the sense of intellectual property) as from a research collaboration with a start-up company.

In the end, the choice of with whom to form a research alliance, or indeed any other kind of partnership, is one that can be taken with the benefit of consideration of the factors included in this book, including financial analyses of net present value or any other method for evaluating worth. The choice is wide, and becoming wider all the time. The vogue quality which currently surrounds partnerships, particularly with the biotechnology sector, permits increasing access to high-quality scientists who have suffered from downsizing within the large companies, or chosen their career in a small company environment. This fashion for such arrangements may have also driven the price of these arrangements to a level that is unacceptably high (see also section 5.2.1.2). If that is the case, small companies may well find the price for their services needs to be reduced to fit a new level of demand. Their continued viability depends on such adaptability.

3.3   LOSS OF CONTROL

Any outside organisation that conducts work for a project that is administered elsewhere is likely to be regarded with at least a modicum of suspicion, sometimes much worse. This partly derives from a 'not-invented-here' reaction which is common in any project, but also includes a strong feeling of lack of trust. Trust in human relationships develops with time, and the very changeability of collaborations which underpins their advantages in terms of flexibility is unlikely to favour trust. All of these factors feed to a greater or lesser extent on loss of control, which is inevitable in a collaborative project.

One of the key elements of preclinical pharmaceutical development is the number and complexity of tasks that must be completed before clinical evaluation can occur. Most of these tasks need to be performed under the charge of highly competent people with decision-making powers. The partnership qualities of the collaborating party have been emphasised before. It is distinctly advantageous that certain decisions of a more tactical nature are taken there.

From this logical sequence of statements, partial control of the project is inevitably passed out from the sponsor to the collaborator. This poses much greater difficulty with regard to management of the developmental programme. In most cases the information available to the project manager is less complete and detailed than would be the case with an in-house project. Collaborators make local decisions more often without recourse to central advice. Conversely, the principle of empowerment at lower levels is a significant component of

Table 3.2 *The need for a balance of control*

Too little control	Too much control
Slippage	Unnecessary extra work by sponsor
Lack of direction	Ineffective use of collaborator's expertise and inventiveness
Poor use of resources	Difficulty in establishing trust
Duplication of effort	

modern management theory. Each time approval for an action is required at a more senior level, delays are incurred. The balance between these factors is a great problem for collaborative projects. The collaborator must be sufficiently empowered to make useful decisions locally, but be sufficiently controlled for the overall smooth running of the entire project (Table 3.2).

With less control, the potential for slippage in a project of a developmental nature is obvious. One reason why this may occur is that the provider has a set of objectives, orthogonal to its clients, of which only some are known to a single sponsor. Providers have to juggle the priorities of different sponsors. Even in the absence of delays for reasons associated with the project at hand, an increase in problems or priority associated with another sponsor's project can have a severe impact.

A sponsor may bring time-related bonus elements to bear to compel or add incentive to the collaborator to meet deadlines. These may only partly address the problem. Delays may still build up for *bona fide* scientific reasons. It is then up to the sponsor to assist resolution or reconfigure other project components to fit a new timescale. In intramural projects, resources may be shifted from one project to another, or one project component to another, according to need. There is less flexibility in doing this when the project is externally contracted, because the associated downgrading in priority of a competing project is not in a sponsor's power. If a sponsor does achieve this, he should recognise the problems that may afflict his competitor sponsor. He may rue the day that he took such action, for he may be on the receiving end too at some time in the future.

The extent to which a sponsor may effectively control an extramural project depends crucially on the quality and quantity of information, and on the advance warning of problems. Similar principles apply to internal projects, but are exacerbated between partners who do not know one another well and who have not developed a trusting relationship.

Loss of control has problems in perception as well as in fact. Slippage and delay are common reasons for decrying the ability of a provider to do his job. The difficulties faced by the provider are often not seen by the sponsor, and even if they are seen, are often poorly understood. Thus the loss of control feeds an incipient mistrust of external agencies. It is interesting to note that such a culture within sponsoring organisations can generate further difficulties with working with collaborators in the future. It is actually very difficult to treat the perceived deficiencies of an external organisation equally to those of an internal department. The whys and wherefores can get lost along the thin corridor of communication that passes through the project co-ordinator, who has a far better opportunity to see that little blame settles on his shoulders.

The comments on control so far have related to developmental projects. They are particularly apt since control is essential for smooth running and timeliness in such projects. In the absence of timeliness, delays can multiply and the whole programme rapidly slips. These aspects are less crucial in research because they do not usually cause multiple, consequential delays. Moreover, any loss of control that may derive from the sponsor can be argued to be compensated by local elements. As described earlier, research collaborations work best where each component feels a sense of ownership, where ideas and motivation are locally bred. Loss of control may equate to a liberating environment that fosters innovation. However, a pharmaceutical research programme without time-based objectives is like a ship without a rudder. True, it may float across sunken treasure, but it is equally likely to drift across rocky shallows, and become holed. Even publicly funded programmes such as those conducted in universities or in governmental research establishments are required to compete with each other under constraints of time-limitation. Such competition, and award of increasingly limited funds, is judged on the basis of track record, and what can be achieved in the next time-limited grant period.

Therefore, the discipline and control of research projects is becoming increasingly tight, whether such projects are conducted in industrial or academic environments. In order to achieve this, successful collaborations require a high degree of cohesiveness and co-operation: this is not always achieved.

3.4   PROBLEMS WITH CROs

The traditional role of the CRO is seen by the organisations themselves as serving the customer. In this role, the maintenance of standards is the key by which CROs feel they are being judged. In so far as they provide data for the successful registration of a product, such standards require rigorous adherence to GLP. CROs have latched onto this criterion as a means of assuring their clients about the quality of the work they do. Such a response is clearly compatible with the client's need to satisfy regulatory bodies, but it is often not compatible with the processes that are required for research. For a start, research requires people to think about what they are doing. The strict adherence to a laid-down protocol that is rarely modified without substantial discussion leaves no room for the normal processes of iteration that accompany drug research. In fact, the attitude of adherence to much earlier-defined protocols is inimical to research, which usually requires a number of trials or tests to be conducted before a definite procedure can be established. For CROs to become important players in pharmaceutical research, as some clearly wish to do, requires a substantial change of philosophy. In a nutshell, although in many cases they are very good at what they do, CROs are really Contract Development Organisations. This is dealt with more substantially in Chapter 5.

CROs' willingness to follow set procedures fits well with a culture that wants direction from the client and defined parameters by which to charge for their services. CROs primarily aim to do a good job for which they are paid, and in satisfying their clients obtain repeat business. In most cases, CROs are unwilling to offer a service at which they feel inexpert; and clients are unwilling to commit significant resources to training CROs to fulfil their needs, when the resultant expertise may be of benefit to competitor companies. For the reasons related to efficiency (see section 2.2) this circuitous situation is not beneficial to the research process. However, it is difficult to see a way out.

For CROs to become true partners in the earlier stages of preclinical drug development and in drug research requires them to risk resources in becoming experts in such areas. They need to anticipate drug companies' requirements in order to be in a position to offer services when they are approached. They need to be able to demonstrate their expertise with data on standard compounds, such data having been acquired at their own expense.

In practice, few CROs are willing to take such risks, since they are perfectly capable of relying exclusively on what they know and are good at. They may be happy to embark on new areas, provided both the learning experience and the data itself are acquired at the expense of the client. Such data may then not be offered to other clients, since rules of confidentiality apply. Rules of confidentiality can pose other problems to CROs. For instance, how should a CRO react to a client's request for a toxicological study on a particular compound based on a mechanistic approach which the CRO has investigated previously for a competitor, and found to possess a mechanism-based side-effect that warranted discontinuation of that therapeutic approach? The answer, in at least one real case, is that the CRO declined to quote for this work, on the basis that the previous experience had been acquired under a confidentiality agreement with another client. This is a rare, perhaps unique case, but emphasises that confidentiality can impede the theoretical efficiency of a common provider.

There is a gap which needs to close between what pharmaceutical companies are willing to pay for CROs to do, and what CROs are willing to risk in developing their business. There are suggestions that a more enlightened era is approaching, and that certain pharmaceutical companies are permitting the transfer of experience gained by a collaborator to competitors. Once such common sourcing is adopted and boundaries of confidentiality more sensibly and loosely defined, the bulk of experience at the CRO that offers such services can make this an even more attractive service to use.

Pfizer's recent research collaboration with Oxford Diversity in the field of combinatorial chemistry was the first of a major company with a provider of this technology in the UK. The initial terms stipulated that Oxford Diversity would be bound solely to Pfizer for two years from the start of the arrangement. In return, Pfizer was making a significant investment and allowing the acquisition of expertise by Oxford Diversity that simply could not have been acquired without its collaboration. However, the terms of the deal were later modified subsequently to permit the smaller company to engage with other pharmaceutical clients before the two year moratorium. As a result of Pfizer's largesse, Oxford Diversity have engaged with a number of other companies as a collaborative partner in combinatorial chemistry.

3.5   PROBLEMS OF ACADEMIC RESEARCH CULTURE

At the other extreme from CROs, many of the contributions from universities to collaborations with the pharmaceutical industry involve a purer adherence to research discipline than is sought by the industry partner. The problems with such an approach can involve a lesser willingness to repeat tried and trusted techniques in favour of continually moving on to newer areas of research. The principles of screening and repetitive evaluation of drugs according to the tests that are warranted by the discovery programme can be difficult to incorporate into a traditional academic–industrial collaboration. Similarly, the 'handle-turning' work that is required for carrying a compound through development is often seen as inappropriately routine for an academic research environment. Academicians prefer, for good reasons of their own, to establish themselves in the scientific community, to push back the frontiers of science rather than consolidate the bridgeheads.

The approach to research work in a university setting is often quite different from that in industry. The goals of the academic are to disseminate his or her results in peer-review journals and books; the work of the industrialist is often published in patents, or submitted for regulatory approval. As most academic research is publicly funded, public dissemination of the results from such endeavours seems to be required. In addition, it is of course necessary for academics to further their careers. This is particularly the case for postgraduate and postdoctoral students. It would be a mistake to insist that all industrially funded academic research should be maintained by the same standards of confidentiality that exist in the pharmaceutical industry.[55] The means of allowing academic research the freedom to publish is one of the key problems for collaborations of this kind, as discussed further in Chapter 4.

Because of the different end-purposes of academic and industrial research, the standards of documentation and record-keeping required for the latter are quite different. It is unlikely, for instance, that GLP is operated in an academic environment. For pharmaceutical research purposes (as opposed to pharmaceutical development), GLP is currently not essential, but increasing formality and detailed quality of reporting is apparent in most pharmaceutical companies, and can be particularly relevant in patent disputes. Since the 1994 GATT accord, the principle of being first to invent, which applied historically to US patents from US notebooks, now applies to notebooks from other countries too; partly as a result of this, good notebooks are now being taken much more seriously in academic circles too. The standards of university record-keeping vary too much to make sweeping statements about their quality. However, if the results of such research are to be integrated into the decision-making process that produces lead compound selection, quality standards are important. A great deal of academic research is conducted by visiting scientists on short-term contracts, and the laboratory records may not be examined in detail until some time after the contract has ended, and the investigator has returned to his native country. This is not to say that deficiency in such records is commonplace; but it certainly can occur. Incomplete documentation can be intensely frustrating, especially when filling in the gaps can require intercontinental telephone calls to the original investigator who has by now returned to a distant land. If experiments need to be repeated, the incumbent delay to the project can be of real disadvantage.

Any collaborative effort with the pharmaceutical industry requires some kind of confidentiality agreement to be in place. Exposure to leaks of confidential information is a problem that by no means besets academic institutions alone, but it is perhaps a greater potential problem there than elsewhere. With research activities, for which academic collaborations are largely used, confidentiality is a particularly evident requirement, since patent cover may well not be complete—indeed there may be none at all if the project has not reached the stage where priority documents can have been filed. Academic institutions are increasingly aware of the advantages of patenting their inventions, but the security arrangements that prevail in the pharmaceutical industry and in CROs are not conducive to the educative role, including free access for students, of academia. The reasons for such security are more to do with the problems of anti-vivisectionist infiltration, and in view of the increasing violence adopted by such people, the principle of free access within academic institutions is likely to become increasingly rare. Moreover, the loss of confidential information of commercial value from a university is more of a theoretical than a real risk. Nevertheless, it remains a concern.

Despite these problems, the appetite for academic collaborations by US industry continues unabated, and in a survey of a number of industrial companies in the life sciences, the extent of such collaboration was expected to increase over the next five years. This expectation applied for both small and large companies including many in the Fortune 500 listing. In addition to the problems associated with confidentiality, academic bureaucracy featured highly among industry responses as a frustration of collaborations.[55]

3.6   TIME AND MOTIVATION

Pharmaceutical R&D in today's competitive climate is a race from start to finish. The product to reach the market first has a great advantage over its successors. In certain circumstances the rapid decision-making qualities of small partners and CROs can offer a time advantage (see section 2.6); but there are pitfalls too. In the first place, management of outsourced activities takes time in itself of the sponsoring company; if the management is thorough, this is certainly not insignificant. Development with qualified in-house resources, with personal relationships built with time on the basis of trust, allows the large pharmaceutical company to burst into a new research project with an immediacy and force that can be very difficult to match in a collaborative arrangement. In a developmental context, project groups will often involve members who have worked together on other projects; the procedures for integrating their roles, for embarking on pieces of work on the basis of phone calls rather than formal instructions, will be in place (or should be in place). Previously pooled experience allows problems to be anticipated before they occur. A well-oiled pharmaceutical development process on one site is difficult to beat provided sufficient resources of the correct kind are devoted, at the right time. In practice this is not always the case, and the international nature of large pharmaceutical companies has made multisite operations commonplace. Moreover, the resources are not just there waiting for the nod to proceed. They are allocated to other projects which need to be prioritised and scheduled in order to afford their maximum utilisation.

Collaborative and even contractual arrangements often take a great deal of time to set up. The complexity of the work, the size of the contract, are both factors that make the arrangements more difficult. The idea of a suitable partner waiting in place for the right piece of work to come along seems implausible, and in practice it is. Such an occurrence would imply inefficiency in the collaborator's business, which runs counter to one of the arguments for contracts and collaborations, namely efficiency (see section 2.2). In reality, contractual work will have to be booked some time in advance, and the management of planned studies (particularly as cancellations can and do occur) is very much part of a CRO's routine. The identification of partner and negotiation prior to any contractual or collaborative piece of work will of course take time in itself. If the aggregate time for negotiation and to find a suitable slot in the contractor's timetable is not adequately allowed for, there will be direct consequential delays. Even if it is allowed for, there are real problems with regard to research activities (which are more difficult to plan), if the lead time is long.

Motivation was mentioned in section 2.5 as an advantage for the collaborative route, on the basis that small companies are more motivated (partly by the fear of failure) than large ones to work hard and achieve results. However, in science in general, motivational impulses are often high anyway. This is particularly so in research where the benefits of successful work accrue to the scientist involved. These benefits include peer group acclaim, or promotion, rather than solely monetary reward. This is the correct reward for ingenuity as much as graft. It has often been said that one cannot have too many good ideas, but the relationship between contracted parties may leave little room for ownership of their own ideas. It is vital that both parties in any collaborative effort feel rewarded for imaginative, positive ideas about how to better achieve the common goal. Janssen has commented that motivation is a prime requirement for successful drug discovery, and that imagination is more important than knowledge.

3.7   GEOGRAPHICAL DISTANCE AND CULTURAL BARRIERS

It need hardly be said that good communication is imperative for successful drug research spanning many disciplines. Collaborative research and development is necessarily more problematic because of geographical dislocation. Regardless of fax and telephone links, and now electronic communication via the Internet, face-to-face contact is necessary too. This is a factor which may be insignificant or it may be impossible. It really depends on the nature of the project: what needs to be done, what resources are available, how competent are the partners at communicating, how tight are the deadlines and how difficult the work is. When Glaxo were persuading the FDA of the need to approve registration of salmeterol, the long-acting β-agonist for asthma, the validity of the clinical data and rationale was communicated by one of their senior clinical representatives; transatlantic flights sometimes twice or thrice a week were called for during the course of negotiations spanning many months. Although the travel was ultimately worth it (at least for Glaxo), and the individual representative has presumably enough air miles to absolve his need ever to purchase another airline ticket, it is an experience that few of us would like to repeat. This is an extreme example, and intensive travel is rarely essential for successful collaborations. Nevertheless, there is a minimum level of travel and face-to-face contact which is necessary, including site visits to the investigator's facilities. It is an added expense to a project, but it is even more a drain on the personnel and their time.

Any operation that involves research on more than one site will need to address technology transfer. In many collaborative efforts, at some time in the process there will be the need to repeat a piece of work at a different site from the one where it was initially performed. Initial efforts will focus on repetition under exactly or closely similar conditions. The validation process is often successful, although detractors of the collaborative approach may point to its inherent inefficiency. The loss of time, duplication of resources and increase in costs are disadvantages which more than offset any advantage from the confidence-enhancing evidence of reproducibility of results. In many cases, the repeat work runs into problems, sometimes for understandable reasons. However, the reasons are sometimes also not understandable in any rational sense, and this is where substantial problems can occur. Chemical reactions often perform differently when operated on a larger scale; pharmacological assays involve a number of factors that can make repetition a more complicated exercise than is apparent at the outset. The reasons for the differences may be unexpectedly trivial, but that very unpredictability can make the cause most difficult to trace. Under these circumstances, partnerships can come under most stress, and questions of proficiency inevitably surface.

Regardless of whether the collaboration is of a research or preclinical development nature, international partnerships can also involve substantial temporal shifts in working time. Collaborations between California and Continental Europe, or Japan and the UK, involve a time difference of 9 hours. For a company such as AMRAD (q.v.) the problems with distance and time zone differences mean that effective collaboration outside of its native Australia is very difficult. The overlap in the normal working day is, in these cases, often non-existent. Allowance for good communication links is also put under strain by differences in public holidays.

Although English is increasingly a *lingua franca*, particularly among the scientific community, communication is difficult between partners of differing mother tongues. Nuances of thought and meaning are often lost, particularly in verbal communication. Resort to the written form can lead to loss of information since one usually has to be sure of what is written: hunches are rarely put down on paper.

In some senses, the very internationality we have come to expect amongst contacts world-wide may obscure the fundamental differences between us. While the global village may in some senses be with us, customs and social behaviour have changed much less rapidly than technology in the past 50 years. What seems polite and correct form in the UK may be very rude in Japan, while it may be overly stiff in the US. Body language, that pseudo-science of the sophomore, is widely different even amongst the Western Europeans. The plan for a common currency in the European Union before the next millennium has produced an intense debate emphasising that we wish to preserve our national identities. The following famous saying may be hackneyed, and not entirely true, but it still strikes a poignant note in the countries it mentions:

> Heaven is where the police are British, the lovers Italian, the cooks French, the engineers German and everything is all organised by the Swiss.

> Hell is where the police are German, the lovers Swiss, the cooks British, the engineers French and everything is all organised by the Italians.

A recent article focused on the problems of this nature faced by international research efforts, particularly as they apply to large multinational companies.[56] These problems also beset extramural collaborations across international barriers of time, culture and language. The above aphorism emphasises that no nation harbours the perfect characteristics in all endeavours. Large projects are increasingly multinational, and where quality personnel are important, this is the more so. The 1996 Formula One racing team from Ferrari was handpicked by a senior executive from the Italian car company Fiat: it comprised a chassis designer from Britain, a Japanese engine builder, a Dutch aerodynamicist, a Swiss development engineer and a French team manager; finally, the car to emerge from this tiger team was driven by a German driver, Michael Schumacher. No doubt they will all communicate in English, but with this many native tongues, one may only ponder in what language they will argue.

Despite advances in communication technology (see section 6.5), there are still problems associated with distance. If the collaboration is at a research stage, samples for biological testing may very well need to be sent across international borders. Unlike fax or electronic communication, physical entities require the intervention of human delivery, which takes time in itself. The preparation of parcels and paperwork to facilitate the delivery are also aspects of tedium and additional labour to that required in a company where the biologist is across the corridor from the chemist who prepared the sample. Another trivial but often important inconvenience is the necessary provision of excess quantities of material in order to assure sufficiency for testing. Occasionally this leads to the requirement for resynthesis which could be obviated without such waste. This is more than inconvenient, since resources will need to be shifted from other tasks.

If the collaboration is of a developmental nature, perhaps to provide material for volunteer studies, then import and export restrictions add an extra level of complexity to the programme. Current regulations in the US restrict use of clinical supplies for human studies to new chemical entities with an IND (Investigational New

Drug) certificate. Volunteer studies in Europe are unencumbered by this bureaucratic restriction and, in the UK, approval of an Ethics committee is required instead. This time advantage is recognised by large pharmaceutical companies and, as a result, 70% of new drug introductions into humans are in Europe; two clinical pharmacology units in the US have recently closed. However, if the raw material manufacture originates in the US, an IND is required for export of any drug intended for human study abroad. In order to bypass this restriction, some additional processing of the material into the final formulation for human use is required.

3.8   CO-ORDINATION AND EXPERTISE

When a project is shifted off-site, more than physical distance separates the two parties. The geographical separation may lead to an intellectual and technological schism. In the extreme case of the so-called virtual research company (see Chapter 6) much of the intellectual expertise is split across sites. Even on a more mundane level, there will be at least two groups working on the same problem from different disciplinary viewpoints. It is the role of a co-ordinator to piece this together to make a gestalt, to assimilate and integrate the results of the outsourced work with other components from in-house efforts. A good co-ordinator must possess an intimate understanding of most if not all of the disciplines that compose the project. Professor Trevor Jones, Director General of the Association of the British Pharmaceutical Industry, has described the essential assets of a project manager (see also section 1.4) as given in Table 3.3.[25a]

Although originally applied for internal projects, these are also the general qualities demanded of a co-ordinator of a number of extramural projects. However, the difficulty for such a person is compounded by the fact that work is conducted on a distant site, and the information received is less often first-hand. When an experiment fails to work in Germany even though the investigator in the UK reported no problems, the most likely reason is that the exact conditions of the experiment were not repeated, based on a failure to communicate all the relevant factors. The deficiency is in the communication, not usually the experimenter. One cannot call all the respective parties to an impromptu meeting down the corridor from their normal workplaces; one cannot see first-hand the working environments, from which the reasons for the discrepancy may appear obvious.

One of the great strengths of the traditional large multinational pharmaceutical company is the tremendous diversity of scientific

Table 3.3   *Requirements of a project manager*

- Omniscient
- Walks on water—and teaches others to do so
- Leaps tall buildings
- Requires no sleep
- An expert in all technical, scientific and clinical areas
- Photographic memory
- Multilingual
- PhD, DSc, MD and MBA
- Circus artist, tightrope walker, juggler, lion tamer, ringmaster, sweeper
- Sober

disciplines and of experience that can be brought to bear on a specific project. That experience, derived from previous projects, is based on analogy which permits experience gained in one area to be readily applied in another. There is a strong element of danger if the process of devolvement is carried too far, and there is insufficient in-house expertise. The gap between the expertise of the internal controllers and the external workers in a project may become quite significant the further the project strays from the scientific background of the former. As the new methods of pharmaceutical R&D become ever-more different it is important that knowledge and experience in a project are not solely to be found in the extramural party. The requirements of the manager of the project in terms of multi-disciplinary talent are not commonly found within the traditional departmental training of the pharmaceutical industry.

If contract and collaborative research and development are to become an increasing component of life in the pharmaceutical industry, there is a need to address the training of entrants to it. The in-depth single-discipline scientific training previously common in large companies may need to be modified for specific personnel whose role will be more project-based. Previous project managers have been able to rely on the wealth of experience of internal scientists. As the reliance on external bodies increases, that body of experience will become less evident. In the extreme, the core of internal managerial personnel who control a particular project may need exceptional multidisciplinary skills. Moreover, the increased level of work performed outside the major organisations will make that very training more, rather than less, difficult. There may come a time when certain aspects of drug development are so routinely carried out by contract that there is a grave lack of expertise left within the sponsor organisation.

One way of dealing with this problem may be to use consultants to bridge the gap between sponsor and CRO. This is another example, on a small scale, of the application of a flexible collaborative arrangement using external resources as a replacement for the traditional permanent employee. However, the difficulties that may occur using skeletal co-ordinating resources are likely to include those occasions when lack of foreknowledge has created a problem that requires substantial rework. In these circumstances, consultants can only help clear up the mess which was created before they arrived.

The multidisciplinary attitude prevalent in large pharmaceutical companies may be very difficult to replicate in collaborative work. True multidisciplinary approaches to a project certainly need to exist at the co-ordinating centre of a network of collaborations. It is necessary to maintain a core of qualified personnel and expertise in-house in order to maintain a minimum amount of directionality, interpretative capability and control. However, in view of what has been said about collaborators participating in the project, it is well that some of that multidisciplinary attitude is conveyed outwards. This may be much easier to achieve in a large pharmaceutical company than in a network of collaborators, some of whom may derive their best work in a single discipline set apart from the context of others. Under these circumstances, it is likely that central control becomes dominant, and collaborators see little in the way of a bigger picture as to the reasons for what they are doing.[57]

Problems of personality become exacerbated in relationships which are more tenuous. The more introverted personality who prefers to wait until the piece of work they are conducting is finished and supported by incontrovertible evidence is ill-suited to such methods of working. These people communicate best through chance, informal encounters at frequent intervals. Voluntary verbal reports, on the basis of incomplete results, are not their style. There may be even worse problems with people who are difficult to control or who are obstinate or inflexible in their attitude to a problem. These types exist in all walks of life, particularly in science and certainly in large companies. But the problems can be ameliorated in environments which require more frequent face-to-face contact. These types of personality present very real problems to collaborative efforts.

3.9 EASE OF CURTAILMENT

There are ups and downs in any pharmaceutical development project. There are many examples of drugs that would not have seen the light of day without the role of a project champion, who has stuck by a perception of the worth of the project despite objective indications of futility. In some cases, senior management has instructed the abandonment of the project, such as was the case with the discovery of the first angiotensin converting enzyme (ACE) inhibitor captopril, sales of which have run into many billions of dollars. Arnold Welch in an autobiographical article[58] describes the history of the discovery of captopril at Squibb. After discovering the potent vasoconstrictor action of the nonapeptide angiotensin II, Welch believed that inhibitors of its production could be beneficial in the treatment of hypertension. Management disagreed, but as Welch describes:[58]

> I was told that the major effort to develop a new and practicable inhibitor of the converting enzyme should be terminated. This, I must state, I refused to do—termination of Welch would have to come first.

As a result of Welch's obstinacy, Ondetti and his collaborators, using the peptides as starting points, synthesised a modified peptide with oral activity, one of a series that later led to the discovery of captopril.[59]

In consequence of this *lèse-majesté*, Squibb have much to be grateful for, but the question arises whether, as a collaborative party, Welch could have done what he did. Surely, the pressure to produce quick results is even greater in such an environment, and the possibility of clandestine research in a smaller company more difficult to engineer. This is the more so because in collaborative arrangements, the costs of the project are that much more visible. Of course, the very visibility and accountability apparent in such projects can be a financial advantage (see section 2.1). Furthermore, the very strength of a project champion can be a disadvantage when the objective analysis suggests strongly that abandonment is advised. On the other hand, the perception of the validity of a scientific approach is more difficult to engender when it is financed by a distant partner. Welch would have had an even harder time in justifying the continuation of the project if he had been part of an extramural research effort. One may only speculate if the ACE inhibitors would have ever arisen in such an environment, or if they could have only been the result of a solely academic research effort.

3.10   INSTABILITY

The problems of instability in outsourced pharmaceutical research and development are much the same as in the engagement of contract construction work, though arguably less severe. Some of the smaller CROs and emerging biotechnology companies tread a fine line between financial rectitude and ruin. Examples of problems ensuing from adverse scientific findings have been cited previously. These, or other events, can severely test the buoyancy of such companies. Those who put their faith in such vehicles for critical-path studies run the risk of events outside their control preventing the completion of the work.

MacroNex is an example of a company that started life in 1990 with founders from Duke University Medical Center, North Carolina, with noble ambitions to discover new treatments for arthritis, athero-sclerosis, cancer and AIDS. A combination of funding from venture capital companies and the US government in the form of a number of Small Business Innovation Research grants (SBIR), totalling around $7m, failed to secure a long-term future for this company. MacroNex formed collaborations with Research Triangle Institute, University of North Carolina, PHYTOpharmaceuticals and Boron Biologicals. It had a clear aim to discover and develop its own therapeutics in collaboration with development partners, although it also offered its proprietary technology, in the form of an *in vitro* assessment of a drug's activity against macrophage function, on a contract basis. Those who availed themselves of this service had to find another source for their requirements beyond mid-1995, when the company ceased to operate. Not only is the business situation often more challenging, but the size of small companies makes them dramatically more dependent on the individuals who are critical to the company's operation. In the case of the virtually organised project involving a number of collaborators, the lean administration of the project means it can become very reliant on individuals, who if they leave can take with them a great deal of expertise specific to the project which can be difficult to replace.

Instability is not a problem that solely affects smaller companies. Recent events have shown that similar problems can affect larger companies too. When two large companies merge or one takes over another, the fusion of the individual companies' research strategies inevitably creates casualties. There may be a knock-on effect concerning collaborations. The formation of Hoechst Marion Roussel in 1995 led to the termination of three collaborations with ImmuLogic, Scios and Alteon, a result of 'reprioritisation of R&D projects'. These companies were left with the option of continuing the research unaided, using their own or further borrowed funds; finding an alternative partner; or discontinuing the work.

To an extent, the problems of instability may be addressed by a suitably foresighted contract at the start of a collaboration. However, this is not a complete solution. Regardless of financial penalties, an incomplete study is an incomplete study. A bankrupt company is by definition a difficult prospect for debt recovery, let alone contractual obligations by way of penalty. Equally, there is increasing evidence, particularly in the US, of merger and acquisition activity amid the burgeoning, but increasingly mature, biotechnology industry. Rather than go directly into receivership, struggling companies may find themselves the subject of unwarranted take-over bids with the aim of stripping assets. They may even find it necessary to solicit such activities, in order to maintain some form of trading; the purchase of Proteus in the UK by ML Laboratories in early 1996 represents an example in which, because of the difficult financial situation in which Proteus found itself, additional funding was necessary and sought from a suitable investor. At the other end of the spectrum, successful companies may also find themselves the target of predatory attention (e.g. Affymax, p. 56), or find other reasons why the current arrangement may not be the best that they can achieve. A significant invention from a collaborator can open the door to applications outside the ambit of the collaborative research, and may suggest to them that alternative avenues are more strategically important than those currently being followed.

The current explosion in new biotechnology start-up companies has created the impression of inexorable growth in this sector. By mid-1996, British Biotech was capitalised at 40% of the value of that of British Steel, the irony magnified by the fact that the latter is one of the most profitable steel operations in the world, whereas the former has yet to pay its shareholders any dividends. The hunger of the large companies for collaborations has created a fertile environment for such ventures. The prospects for future growth are good, but the current pace of growth cannot continue forever. At some point the biotechnology sector will mature, and subsequently there will be a period of consolidation. The less secure, the less well run, and the less fortunate will fall; the others may well prosper. *Caveat emptor*—let the buyer beware.

4
The Role of Academic Institutes

4.1 INTRODUCTION

The nature of the interactions between industry in general, and the pharmaceutical industry in particular, and the universities has changed significantly during the last two decades. A substantial restructuring of the public sector research base, which includes government laboratories and research institutions as well as the universities, has occurred. These changes continue to be driven by a number of factors. Foremost among these is the recognition that, while universities carry out a substantial proportion of the basic research carried out nationally and internationally, improvements are needed in the processes whereby the economic potential of the results of that research is realised.

Legislative changes in the US and the UK have allowed universities to own and exploit their own intellectual property. In the biotechnology sector, the Nobel prize-winning discovery by Cohen and Boyer that DNA can be cut, recombined and inserted into foreign bacteria has opened up a new dimension in molecular biology which has led to the rapid growth of the biotechnology industry. Biotechnology has had a major impact on the way that traditional pharmaceutical research is carried out and currently is leading to the production of biologically derived therapeutic agents in its own right. The mutual interactions between industry and the US universities in this sector have been well described in Kenney's book[60] and a more mechanistic analysis of linkages between the two sectors with a European focus in the book by Konecny et al.[61]

In the US notably, the relative proportions of university and industrial basic research have shifted dramatically since the end of the Second World War.[62] This trend is likely to continue, at least in Western economies, as more and more companies are closing down their central research facilities with the objective of creating leaner organisations, generating greater shareholder value, at least in the short term. In the pharmaceutical sector, the current wave of amalgamations and take-overs amongst the major companies has also resulted in a total decrease in research activity and may have reduced the overall chances of innovative research being carried out in-house. Every organisation has its own ethos and approach to research and the greater the variety of approaches to solving a problem the greater the chance of genuine innovation.

Outside the pharmaceutical sector, companies have chosen to close their central facilities largely on the grounds that research is very expensive, the results by their very nature unpredictable and the value of the linkages between research and the sale of products, long term, tenuous and hard to quantify. The return on research investment is not capable of simple analysis in the short term, and is difficult to quantify even in the long term. Paradoxically, it is increasingly recognised that it is fundamental research which supplies the seed corn results for the products of tomorrow, but, if the decision is made to reduce in-house research, those results must of necessity ultimately be obtained from work carried out elsewhere. They must both be accessible and in a form capable of being integrated into a company's business. Implicit in the closure of central facilities is the recognition of the inadequacy of the links between the activities of the central facilities and those of the operating divisions, and the mutual failure of each to perceive their reciprocal value and to integrate their activities. If it is difficult to sustain and realise the value of such links internally, it is even more difficult to achieve this externally, and this is an absolutely crucial factor to bear in mind when contemplating collaborations with universities, and substituting a physical with a virtual research company.

As a result of the general decrease in industrial research activity, universities increasingly play a key role in carrying out basic research within the economy. In addition to his/her intellectual talents, the academic scientist enjoys a number of other advantages in providing services to industry. These include:

• access to good scientific facilities
• access to willing student labour
• library and information facilities
• aptitude to work and collaborate with external bodies
• multidisciplinary colleagues

Governments from whence universities obtain their funding are also subject to economic pressures, and like industry, in the face of a fiercely competitive global economy, wrestle with the questions of how much to spend on research, how to assess the value of research and how to maximise the benefits that result. Western governments, notably in the UK and the US, are currently trying hard to limit severely the amount spent on basic research in universities. In contrast, Japan and the Tiger economies of the Pacific rim give a higher priority to long-term research and are increasing their research spending, perhaps partly as a reaction to the Western stance. The dynamic tensions that exist between the supporters of either industrial or government funding of basic research are well described in Kealey's controversial book.[63]

Despite the surprising persistence of the belief that all research in universities is nothing but 'blue skies' and seeks only to provide descriptions and explanations of the structure and function of the physical universe, contacts, and the transfer of research results, between universities and industry have a long and successful history. As so often, simple generalisations rapidly crumble when subjected to detailed analysis. The genesis of the German and British dyestuffs industry in the nineteenth century resulted from research carried out in university laboratories and, in this century, the rapid growth of the computer, electronics, synthetic materials and pharmaceutical industries has been based on scientific theories and discoveries and a reciprocal relationship between these industries and the science base. In the USA, the land grant universities were set up in the last century with public funds to address the needs of the agricultural production system (food and fibre, especially cotton), an example of the market dictating the focus of government initiative in the academic sector. This was followed on by new programmes in engineering, mining and metallurgy in the early part of this century; examples of such universities that are active in the biotechnology sector include UC Berkeley, UC Davis, Wisconsin, Cornell and Minnesota. It can be argued that university departments of, for example, computer science, engineering and medicine would not exist in their current form, if at all, were there not associated industries and professions to employ the graduates and use the research results that these departments produce. Conversely such industries often provide the challenging long-term problems which are the feedstock of academic research.

Links with the pharmaceutical industry currently have the highest profile as they are the best financed, because of the research intensity of the industry and the explosive growth of the biotechnology sector. Such linkages are not surprising and reflect the value that this sector places on innovation and therapeutic advances, its constant need for new research personnel and its understanding of the high risks and the long timescales involved in turning the results of research into successful products. The industry has to some extent even educated its shareholders and financial analysts with regard to this fact. The well-documented phases of drug development contrast with the development of many other consumer products and provide an explicit yardstick by which a company's progress may be measured by its investors, its analysts and its own managers. Even so, the difficulty of valuing preclinical research remains a permanent problem as, by its very nature, the outcomes are highly uncertain.

Industry and universities are therefore focusing at a strategic level on the value and mutual benefits to be obtained from collaboration. For industry the benefits include access to current research results as potential new sources of innovation which, in turn, lead to technical and commercial advantage in the marketplace, access to high-quality collaborators, access to future graduate and postgraduate employees and access to unique equipment, facilities and libraries. Universities clearly benefit, as immediate funding increases their resources which may, in turn, attract further public funding. Commercial, market-based insights provide new perspectives and dimensions for academic research and industry's task-orientated approach to problem solving frequently stimulates highly productive multidisciplinary collaborations. There are many mechanisms for collaboration, making simple generalisations impossible. The nature and success of relationships vary from industry to industry, from company to company, from university to university and from individual to individual within these organisations. The need for effective links between the industrial and academic sectors has therefore never been more crucial if the overall economic rewards are to be realised from the research investment made in both. This topic has been the subject of a UK Government White Paper, the first on this subject for over twenty years.[64] It is necessary, therefore, to consider the nature of the academic sector, the nature of its links with the pharmaceutical industry and how the potential value of these links may be realised.

4.2   THE NATURE OF UNIVERSITIES

The *Concise Oxford Dictionary* defines a university as an 'educational institute designed for the instruction or examination or both of students in all or many of the more important branches of advanced learning, conferring degrees in various faculties, and often embodying colleges and similar institutions'. Interestingly, this definition makes no mention of research and, for anyone unfamiliar with the Oxbridge systems, the reference to colleges is somewhat gratuitous. Gordon Johnson in his book *University Politics*[65] describes the University of Cambridge as 'one of those peculiar forms of social organisation which have evolved for the express purpose of creating, discovering, preserving and transmitting knowledge'; this is a more helpful description that may be applied to all universities although clearly some are more peculiar than others. Irrespective of the definition, the core business of universities is teaching and research, they operate on a long timescale and history at least suggests that, as organisations, they may well outlast the companies if indeed not the industries with which they currently collaborate.

The prime teaching task of universities is to provide society with well-educated and well-trained people who are capable not only of creating new knowledge but also, and importantly, of assimilating and applying existing knowledge to new problems and challenges. Universities therefore have a critical role in supplying the pharmaceutical industry with the scientific and engineering personnel that it needs. The rapid changes in the infrastructure of this industry have forced an increased awareness of the personal attributes needed in its employees. The number of jobs, in relationship to the number of scientific degrees awarded, is declining, itself providing negative feedback to anyone considering a scientific career. At the same time the need for exceptionally able people to cope with the enormous challenges of a changing industry has never been greater. While the industry generally recruits doctoral level scientists into its research laboratories, it is clear that the traditional research-based training of these scientists is inadequate and what has been called 'parascientific' training[66] in, for example, technology transfer in a broad sense, management, legal and commercial issues are now needed to enable such employees to operate successfully in an increasingly complex multidisciplinary environment. Given the restructuring of the industry, the prospect of a career for life within a single company is no longer realistic.

Research in universities is largely carried out by postgraduate students and postdoctoral researchers supervised by the permanent faculty. The latter spend increasing amounts of time raising funds to support the former and the balance between permanent staff and those supported on so-called soft money has changed so that workers on short-term contracts greatly outnumber permanent members of staff. Funding is obtained from an increasing variety of sources including from the state, from industry and, notably in the biomedical sector, from the major medical charities of which The Wellcome Trust, consequent to the sale of its shares in Wellcome plc to Glaxo, is now the largest medical charity in the world. It is notable that in the biomedical area of research in UK universities, the ratio of public to private funding is about 1:1 compared with 3:1 in the biological sciences and 4.6:1 in the non-bioscience area.[67]

The cost of carrying out research has increased enormously, especially in the area of molecular biology, and the demand for resources from the traditional sources of the state and the charities substantially outstrips the supply. Increasingly, researchers are looking to industry for support for basic research, and this is inevitably leading to new arrangements and relationships being established.

Research in universities serves a dual function in that new researchers receive training while working at the frontiers of knowledge, while research in industry is carried out with the aim of producing new products and processes. The importance of the movement of these individuals as a means of transferring scientific and technical knowledge into industry cannot be over-emphasised and is arguably the most effective vehicle for the transfer of such knowledge into industry. The results of academic research are normally disseminated by oral presentations at conferences and the like and by written publications in the open scientific literature. Electronic forms of communication are increasingly playing a role and while they have facilitated global collaboration, they have at the same time increased both the pace of research, and also the level of competition. The ability to keep up on an essentially instantaneous basis with the activities of both collaborators and competitors globally has become routine for most academic scientists. The academic community is networked internationally in a way that many companies have yet to achieve or in some cases even to imagine. The openness of the academic community lends itself to such forms of communication and contrasts with the need for confidentiality in commercial communications. Industry is understandably concerned with confidentiality although it has been observed that security breaches usually occur internally and by leakage and not by external infiltration. Excessive confidentiality conversely often leads to mistrust and results in valuable information being rendered unavailable at the expense of the information that is protected.

4.3   CURRENT PATTERNS OF LINKAGE

Research and development activity and links with universities in the pharmaceutical industry is a post-war phenomenon. Before the Second World War, the pharmaceutical industry mainly produced commodity products in the form of active ingredients which were turned into final products by the retail pharmacies. The costs of active ingredients as a proportion of the products were high and the industry spent little on research and development. In the Second World War, research for a cure for malaria and other tropical diseases, and on the large-scale production of penicillin in the US, led in the 1950s to the evolution of pharmaceutical companies that combined the manufacture of raw materials, drug research, manufacture and marketing. The production of penicillin was driven by a crucial need for a means of treating septicaemia in the wounded of the Second World War, but was made possible by Sir Alexander Fleming's fundamental observations on bacterial growth at St Mary's Hospital in London, many years previously in 1928. As the industry developed, the costs of drugs as a proportion of the costs of products started to fall, and by the 1960s the need for innovation had become critical in order for companies continually to produce new drugs as old ones dropped out of patent protection. This was essential to maintain let alone increase their share of the market. By this time, the cost of R&D increased to some 8% of the cost of sales, and has increased further so that today the pharmaceutical industry is research intensive compared with virtually all other industries and spends more on R&D than any other single form of investment.

Universities provided the industry with employees and consultancy but pursued their research and their search for scientific truths largely unconnected with the needs of the marketplace and continued to publish the results of their research in the open literature. Such funds as industry supplied were often on a donation basis, were undirected and had few strings attached. They were sometimes regarded as a form of duty rather than an activity which might affect the bottom line. Research funds were relatively plentiful, the university system was expanding and, hard as it is to believe now, academic salaries were competitive or even ahead of those offered by industry. Science policy was guided by the idea of a linear process starting with fundamental research in universities which somehow was translated into technology and as a result of industrial development yielded new products for the market.

With the 1970s came the general economic downturn, university budgets became increasingly squeezed by governments, and industry increasingly focused on shorter term objectives. The need for better links between the publicly funded science base and the industrial sector for their mutual advantage, and in order for government to justify better the sums expended, became more explicit. Most universities now have business development departments (or industrial liaison offices), to exploit their inventions, and patent offices to protect them. There are now directories which list the activities of various university departments, and even individual groups of investigators. This information can be obtained from the university liaison offices themselves, in some cases through the information present on their World Wide Web home pages. More centralised directories are also available, such as that published in the UK by Oakland Consultancy in Cambridge.[54] The drive for academic collaboration has also come from industry, and in the 1980s there was a pronounced response to the appeal of rational drug design and the success of basic scientific research as exemplified by the Nobel laureate Sir James Black. At the same time the linear model of innovation has been gradually discarded as it is now recognised that market pull and the needs of customers also shape the course of science. New products are frequently based on incremental improvements on the old, and technology itself promotes the need to understand better the underpinning science. Contact with industry is seen as an opportunity, not a chore. With it, the acceptability of applied science is growing. The aim is more for the improved application of scientific developments for the benefit of humankind, not for the achievement of scientific discoveries *per se*.

Part of the shift has derived from the restrictions on university funding. Grants councils are increasingly viewing industrial collaboration as an indication of sanction of quality, as well as of applicability and relevance. In the UK, university departments are rated by the Higher Education Funding Councils. The rating they receive depends in part on the degree to which they can attract industrial funding. Such funding indicates the relevance of their work to the real world, in addition to vouching for its quality in an alternative way to academic peer review.

Interestingly, biotechnology does provide an example of the linear model of research in that the key discoveries of the structure of DNA, the production of monoclonal antibodies, and recombinant techniques all took place in an academic environment. It is still the case that the academic sector, with a few notable exceptions such as the invention of the polymerase chain reaction by Kary Mullis at Cetus, is producing the fundamental research on which the industry is based. Current research on the human genome falls into an interesting category in that it is fundamental but it is being promoted vigorously and supported by both the public and private sectors as a result of the potential medical and commercial uses to which the results might be put. The well-documented controversies over the patenting of the results of research in this area have highlighted very vividly the tensions engendered by the conflicts arising from the need and wish of academic scientists to put the results of their work into the public domain and industry's need to preserve its competitive advantage by protecting its position. This is a key issue in academic–industry relationships and will be returned to later.

Where the financial involvement is in the form of a grant, industry rarely achieves the complete devotion of the academic through its funding. Industry normally recognises this, and usually does not expect 100% of a student's or technician's time and effort. For real benefit to be gained from industrial–academic collaborations, there needs to be a commitment on both sides for results to be achieved, which can be jointly interpreted as useful. In other words, both sides need the same agenda. This can be arranged by allocating percentages of time that will be spent pursuing 'pure' and 'applied' research goals. Such percentages may usually be incorporated in a mutual unwritten understanding between academic and industrial supervisors. However, as time goes by there can be a tendency for the local management to predominate. On the other hand, to fix the relative proportions in the form of a written contract would be difficult to enforce without controls that would be unlikely to work in an academic setting; furthermore, such controls would be counterproductive because of the ill-feeling they would generate. A flexible approach has much to recommend it, in which both sides appreciate the priorities of the other.

Industrialists often profess that academics have a poor understanding of deadlines and schedules. A more accurate statement would assert that academics often have a less than full commitment to the industrialist's deadlines. One problem lies in poor communication between the two partners as to what is required and when, and what priorities to afford to what. Another is that the incentives for the collaboration to work are not sufficiently shared.

The best collaborative exercises derive from rapidly growing and changing fields. In these, industry may have an incomplete understanding of the scope of the practical possibilities, but wishes to find them out. Academic collaborations can move forward the boundaries of the science in a 'pure' way while allowing the partnership to offer the industrial sponsor first-hand access to the emerging technology. In such cases, the academic can be left a free hand to pursue his or her perceived best way forward. The concept of parallel industrial and academic objectives is not necessary; both have the same goal.

It is often in the interests of both sides for the collaboration to exist for two to three years, which is commensurate with the timespan of a postdoctoral or PhD studentship. Some collaborations, particularly with Japanese sponsors, are inclined to be for longer periods, up to five to ten years. Supporters of 'basic' research collaborations might find this better for work with less immediate horizons. Overall productivity on very short timescales is diminished because of the inevitable 'setting-up' period, which makes such arrangements less desirable. Long periods may not suit the increasing flexibility that industry really wants; nor does it suit the situation in which the person who set the collaboration up in the first place has moved company or been promoted within a company and a new supervisor appears. In addition to the tendency for long-term collaborations to become 'stale', such arrangements also tend to become rather rigid. The two to three year period is commensurate with the time period of a successful drug discovery project—i.e. prior to entry into preclinical development. Nevertheless, there are undoubtedly instances where great success has been achieved over longer periods of time. For example, SmithKline Beecham has supported the University of Cambridge Department of Medicine since 1987, but not in a focused way, involving targeted drug research. Instead the funding has been directed both at the Department, for laboratory equipment, and in a generic way at the research carried on within, in the form of grants which are applied for internally. The benefits of this system to SB presumably derive from intangible elements related to good relationships with the university and access to potential employees emanating from the department.

Traditionally, collaborations and ultimately the transfer of technology have been established largely by *ad hoc* processes driven by the personal enthusiasms of individuals and often by their geographical proximity. Consultancies undertaken by individual members of university staff for governments, charities and for industry are a traditional form of interaction with external agencies and a further way of externalising the results of research. Most universities encourage consultancy, or at least do not actively discourage it, and see it as having a beneficial impact on both research and teaching, as well as providing a beneficial service to industry and the other agencies and providing additional income to faculty members. In the UK at least, academic salaries are exceedingly uncompetitive at present, and in certain areas of science, the freedom for individuals to be able to carry out consultancy is essential if the universities are to attract and retain the services of high-calibre personnel. Inevitably there are major and difficult issues of personal accountability and potentially substantial conflicts of interest between maintaining a teaching programme and a research group, while at the same time performing confidential work for industry, especially if that industry is one in which the academic has a personal interest. This area is fraught with difficulties and any attempts to police it in a heavy-handed way either drive it underground or destroy the demonstrable benefits. In light of the huge expansion of the biotechnology-based sector, and their massive current dependence on the output of university research and access to faculty members as consultants and/or members of their scientific advisory boards, it is clear that new guidelines and norms of behaviour will need to be established and accommodated.

Consultancy provides a company with state of the art information and also provides a means of obtaining access to potential employees. In addition it often leads to further collaborative research work within the consultant's research group. Consultancies are generally established by personal contacts between companies and individuals who are often identified on the basis of their published work or increasingly by an active process facilitated by university companies established for that purpose or by the universities' own industrial liaison offices (ILOs). The use of consultants can be very cost-effective to a company as it provides an effective gateway to the global network of academic scientists and may be more economical than employing in-house staff for keeping abreast of current developments. Consultants may be used for advice on specific technical issues or for more strategic purposes. In either case it is important that companies seek the best available advice from the most appropriate source regardless of their physical location.

To promote collaboration, a number of public sector mechanisms have been set up to stimulate the contact between industry and the publicly funded science base. One of the oldest in the UK is the CASE scheme (Co-operative Awards in Science and Engineering) which was set up in the late 1960s by the Science Research Council (SRC). This is a scheme whereby postgraduate students receive a grant from the SRC which is supplemented by a contribution from a collaborating company. The student has an industrial supervisor as well as an academic supervisor and spends some time during their studentship working on the company's premises. Nominally the project would have a practical purpose in solving a problem that industry either wanted or thought that it would be worthwhile to solve. The scheme was conceived as a way of pump-priming a process that would lead to more strategic and substantial collaborations. Even in the pharmaceutical sector, initially such studentships were regarded rather snobbishly as being less attractive than the normal form of research grant as if they were somehow contaminated by the industrial component, reflecting the very disjunction between the two sectors that this scheme was hoping to remove.

The scheme has successfully survived the test of time and today is generally popular both with students and their supervisors. It provides students with an enhanced level of income compared with a normal grant and generally the contact with industry is well regarded even though the actual research content of the collaboration is often of marginal interest to the company. Detractors of the scheme have argued that the value of the research to industry is very low, as reflected in the level of direct funding that is provided, although often overlooked is the substantial opportunity cost to the industry itself in setting up, administering the scheme and playing host to the student. If the problem was of burning importance, it would have been totally industrially funded. From the industrialist's point of view, much of the benefit was derived from the advance awareness of the student's capabilities (which, given the inadequacies of the selection process defined above, are not insubstantial—see section 2.4.2), and from the consultative advice that could be gained from contact with the academic supervisor. In addition, the scheme has brought the two sectors together over and above the interaction derived from a conventional studentship. In summary, the scheme is an excellent way of establishing an initial contact between a company and a research worker, but in some ways it raised false expectations in some quarters, as the value to industry of the research produced was misconceived.

In fact, discoveries emanating from CASE collaborations that have become of great worth have presented a problem. If the industrial partner wishes to protect the invention and file a patent or patents, the PhD thesis is often presented to the university and published *in camera*, under which public disclosure can be delayed indefinitely. While this has happened in a number of cases, by and large the CASE system has not greatly pushed forward the research activities of pharmaceutical companies. In consequence there may have been a tendency by some to see all industrial involvement with academic research as a rather self-indulgent exercise. This is incorrect, and other models of industrial–academic collaboration have been more fruitful.

A more substantially funded and focused programme for post-graduates is the Teaching Company Scheme, based on the analogy of a teaching hospital, whereby a recently graduated student works within a company for one or two years on a specific project. The work is again jointly supervised by an academic supervisor in the collaborating university and by an industrial supervisor. The student, known as a Teaching Company Associate, usually registers for a masters degree with the associated university and receives training suitable for an industry-based career. The scheme requires a considerable investment of time and money by all parties but has proved very successful, provided the company is able to disseminate the knowledge generated internally. Frequently the students working on the scheme join their host company as employees, and clear financial benefits to the sponsoring companies' performance have now been documented. The scheme is funded by various public sector bodies including the Department of Trade and Industry (DTI) and a number of the research councils, with a matching contribution from the company. It is largely centred on the engineering sector, as it was perceived this was where enhanced technical and managerial skills and increased investments in training, research and development were needed. Recently a number of programmes have been set up in the biotechnology sector with every expectation of comparable success. The effectiveness of the scheme has been recently assessed.[68]

In contrast to the student-centred programmes are the LINK programmes set up in the late 1980s with the explicit aim of increasing the benefits to the UK economy of the public investment in science. Their objectives were to foster priority areas of scientific research and stimulate investment directed towards the development of innovative services, processes and products, to improve the links between the public and private sector research base, and to develop technologies that crossed disciplinary and sectoral boundaries. The basis of the scheme was the formation of consortia which included a number of companies and institutions working in strategic areas of research. The consortia were funded half by public money and half by industry. The selected areas of research are described for political reasons as pre-competitive but at the same time are intended to have significant prospects of commercial relevance and the industrial parties should be capable of exploiting the results.

Initially a group of companies was required to work together but the scheme was soon modified to allow one-to-one collaborations. Nearly fifty programmes have been run to date of which about a third have been, or are, in the biomedical arena or biotechnology, but relatively few have been explicitly aimed at the pharmaceutical sector except specific programmes on drug delivery and asymmetric synthesis. The LINK programmes are conceptually similar in many ways to the EU Framework Programmes set up originally in the mid-1980s. These are more explicitly focused in areas where Europe as a whole was deemed to be technically deficient and where the stimulation of transnational collaboration, and the education and movement of young researchers are perceived as crucial to the establishment of the unified market. Once again the emphasis is on generic biotechnology and healthcare in a broad sense rather than research specifically orientated towards the pharmaceutical sector.

The need for public sector intervention or for pump-priming funds has been much less evident in the pharmaceutical sector and is reflected in the 1:1 ratio of public to private funding mentioned earlier. Collaborative research arrangements set up directly between the industry and individual members of the academic staff of universities, without a direct contribution from the public sector, are the norm, although CASE studentships are widespread and the scheme has always been well supported by the major pharmaceutical companies. The conventional pattern is for the company to fund fully a studentship, or to pay the direct costs of a postdoctoral research fellow to work in an area of mutual interest to the company and the faculty member. These arrangements are generally brought about by the same mechanisms as consultancies, i.e. by direct contact between the company and the member of staff as a result of mutual knowledge of each other's activities, and by use of intermediaries including the ILOs. They may also result from contacts established initially via consultancies and frequently involve an active consultancy input from the academic staff member paid, in some cases, in the form of a retainer.

As has been mentioned, the traditional nature of the interactions has been informal and established by *ad hoc* processes such as meetings at conferences and other personal contacts. As the links have become more formal and the pressure on universities to diversify their sources of income has increased greatly, collaborations are becoming enmeshed in complex contractual issues. Issues such as costing and pricing of research, overhead recovery, conflicts of interest, publications and the ownership of intellectual property generated from collaborations have to be addressed seriously and professionally. If they are not managed effectively, major disincentives to collaboration will occur ultimately to the detriment of all parties. From the perspective of the UK, companies that recognise and value collaboration can react to poorly managed collaborations by initiating in-house research or by seeking partners in Continental Europe, in the USA or in the rapidly expanding Pacific rim economies. The latter are investing heavily in training and research, notably in areas of biotechnology of potential direct relevance to the pharmaceutical industry. The competitive element to attracting industrial collaborations applies internationally, particularly for companies that have a world-wide presence, and countries other than the UK also recognise this.

Most basic research in universities does not produce results of immediate commercial value and is not driven by market-led imperatives. The belief that universities are sitting on undiscovered pots of gold or are technological sleeping beauties, merely awaiting the awakening kiss of a handsome financier, still lingers in some quarters, although it is generally taken for granted that the value of the outputs of universities is not fully realised and that more can be extracted. The argument that as industry recognises the value of long-term research in universities it will be prepared to pay for it, is at odds with the current emphasis on increasing shareholder value in the short term. Conversely, cuts by the government in university funding have been met by suggestions from the financial sector that all the universities need to do is to exploit better their own research results to generate income to make up the shortfalls. Why universities should be better placed to do this than industry, and how they might achieve this objective, is not explained.

4.4   CONTRACTUAL ISSUES

The costing and pricing of academic research is a complex issue. Universities engage in a diversity of activities and receive funds from a variety of sources. Attributing the use of these financial resources to particular activities in the face of this diversity is extremely difficult. Teaching and research are the core activities, both in the UK and abroad, and are regarded as inseparable and mutually beneficial. In the UK and the US, universities are classified as charitable or not-for-profit organisations, and in order to retain the benefits of such status, are not allowed to trade or to use the resources they receive from the public purse to subsidise directly industrial activities. In Europe strict anti-competition rules apply to public–private sector interactions permitting no more than equal funding of collaborative projects by each sector. The need to address these issues is essential particularly in the face of an increasing squeeze on university resources, a continuing need to diversify the sources of funding and a need to retain the quality of output in the face of an increasing demand.

Universities often have unique facilities and the ability to generate unattributed income from their exploitation is both superficially attractive and potentially valuable, but universities need to consider the opportunity costs of carrying out such work, and recognise that normal commercial forces apply. A useful distinction exists between the collaborative exercises by contract research organisations and those by academia with the pharmaceutical industry. The former exist solely to serve their clients, whereas the latter use these relationships to enable them to better serve their main purpose, which is as institutions that educate and advance knowledge. Contracts whereby a university carries out a piece of work such as the bioassay or spectroscopic analysis of compounds, or clinical trials, the results of which are confidential to the company, are of the same type as a CRO might provide. If a university seeks to emulate a contract research laboratory, it must behave in a business-like way, and of course any company considering such work must consider the cost, alongside the benefit of carrying it out in an open university environment. Proper costing and pricing of such work should remove the potential for undercutting commercial competitors on the basis of a hidden subsidy from the public purse, but exposes universities to the potentially difficult area of trading for profit, a conflict of interest with the charitable objectives of the university. This can be avoided by using a company set up for the purpose of managing such activities, and which can return its profits in a tax-effective manner to the university, via a covenant or by deed of gift. Generation of income is a clear motivating factor but more fundamental are the issues of why the university should engage in such activities in the first place, the ultimate impact on its core business, and whether this is consistent with its own long-term objectives.

These issues aside, such purely commercial contracts are conceptually straightforward. More common but more complex to negotiate and establish are collaborative contracts. In a successful and genuine collaboration all parties should be interested in, and committed to, carrying out the work. All parties should be interested in the output and, in principle, all parties should benefit from the output if it is of commercial value. Costing, pricing, attribution of resources and dealing with the intellectual property rights are vital if such arrangements are to work successfully. The CASE scheme illustrates this point well, being one of the longest-running collaborative schemes. It is rightly popular with researchers, but has occasionally led to difficult negotiations between company lawyers and university administrators. The researchers on each side are generally well aware of the realities of the potential commercial value of the research that results. However, some company lawyers—sometimes aided by, but often out of touch with, the scientific managers of the programmes—have necessarily assumed that the outcomes will be of substantial commercial value, and treated the contract as if it was a contract with another commercial organisation. Attempts have been made to impose difficult if not impossible publication arrangements, and industrial ownership of all the output has been insisted on, with no return to the university, despite the low level of their company's financial contributions. University administrators have reacted accordingly, and this has provoked levels of acrimonious exchanges out of all proportion to the financial inputs and intellectual outputs of the schemes, the real benefits and purposes of the programme having been completely forgotten.

The mechanism by which UK universities receive funding from the government, and the intimate intermingling of research and teaching, has inadvertently but effectively kept both academics and industrialists in blissful ignorance of the real costs to the universities of carrying out research. Now that universities are being forced to consider these issues very seriously, it has become very apparent that there was a substantial level of cross-subsidy between these activities. For effective financial management, the existence of these subsidies must be recognised and either explicitly tolerated for strategic reasons or eliminated.

The budget of a collaborative agreement usually consists of a relatively few components namely staff costs, consumable items, travel, equipment, possibly a contingency element, and an appropriate level of overhead normally stated as a percentage of staff costs. The last item is the most difficult to quantify and is the cause of substantial disagreements between universities and companies in recent years. It is the most intangible and variable item in a budget and, as a result, is generally regarded as negotiable, despite the fact that overheads are real costs and not some form of optional profit.

Research grants from the UK Research Councils to British universities by contracts with all forms of industry amounted to £122m in 1993–4.[69] On average, this is a contribution to university overheads of 43% on the salary component. A figure of 40% as an overhead in academic collaborations is regarded as standard in some circles, although the origin of this figure is obscure and the route by which this income reached the university even more so. This situation has changed, and Research Council grants now bring with them at least some of their associated overhead. For instance, the normal rate for the constituent colleges of the University of London is 40–60%, but other institutions may charge substantially more or less. A recent analysis has revealed the extent to which this was an underestimate, particularly as it fails to take into account the overhead associated with the time an academic supervisor spends on a project, or the costs of the buildings in which the work is housed. Nevertheless this figure has become enshrined in UK university and industry folklore. It is still perceived in both quarters as being a real figure, and therefore acceptable or even excessive, despite industry's knowledge that its own overheads are very much higher. The 'true' overhead figure has been estimated as high as 100–150%. The fair rate of overhead is a difficult figure to arrive at. Academic administrators, mindful of the widespread financial difficulties faced in academic institutions, argue that industry is paying too little. From the industry side, there is also a minority view, fortunately less prevalent in the pharmaceutical sector, that since universities are funded from the public purse and since companies pay corporation tax, the services of universities should be available essentially free of charge. Notwithstanding the fact that corporation tax is a relatively small component of the income received by the government, this attitude to universities is hardly consistent with the realities of life. It can only be assumed that the individuals making such remarks pay neither postage nor road tax and were used to travelling free on British Rail.

The overhead rate depends on the institution, the nature of the work (i.e. the extent to which it facilitates or overlaps with ongoing academic research) and the magnitude of the collaboration. There are wide variations. The final figure may be negotiable. In addition to prowess, which can be quantified in terms of ratings from the Department of Education, there are other factors of a rather more fickle nature which can govern the overhead percentage. There is little concept of a market rate for these charges.

In a traditional collaboration with industry, the difficulty for the academician, as always, is balancing the collaborative role with that of his primary purpose, which is normally an educational one. It is important that the resources committed to a collaboration are used for the purpose intended, but because of the multifunctional nature of the university environment, there is always the suspicion by industry that overheads are being misappropriated to support infrastructure unrelated to the project. At the same time, some well-known academics tread a fine line in using university facilities for commercial purposes. Facilities related to teaching are the prime suspect but the playing fields, catering and, in a celebrated case in the USA, the President's yacht (and his wife's flowers), are among others. Strangely, the academic who has worked hard to attract such support sees none of the overhead portion of the financial contribution, nor does s/he have any say in setting it. Industry sometimes finds itself on the same side as the individual academic investigator, who is anxious to benefit from external funding, intellectually motivated by the science, and set to derive little or no benefit from the overhead rate which sinks, unrecoverably, into the red leather furbishments of the Rector's office. Thus it is unfortunately possible for industry and academics to conspire together to undermine the financial health of the organisation in which the research takes place. Once universities are better able to estimate effectively the costs associated with research, they will be in a stronger position to calculate the price that industry might be expected to pay for collaborative activities, to justify that price from a position of authority and to render the whole process more transparent to all the potential beneficiaries. Industry, understandably, will wish to contain costs, particularly as industrial budgets for collaboration are increasingly being devolved to the operating level rather than centrally awarded, and in the short term if university prices rise, a reduction in the total volume of collaborative research might be expected to result. In the longer term, provided the parties are truly committed to the association, the system will recover, as universities have unique resources and capabilities which they are trying to exploit. If this is not the case then industry always has the choice of doing the work in-house, finding an alternative source or, of course, of not doing the work at all.

It is sometimes argued that there is an open market for research in universities and that they can compete with each other on price. This may be true for contract research, but in general academic scientists compete for their primary research funds from the same national sources, and at the same national rates. It would be rare for funding bodies to award grants for identical work in different locations and, as a result, research in different groups tends to be highly individual and complementary in nature, rather than directly competitive, and therefore in a specified area, industry may actually be limited in the choice of individuals with whom it would wish to collaborate. Conversely, if individuals are working in a very fashionable field such as, currently, combinatorial chemistry, they may be faced with the difficult task of choosing between different sponsors if it proves not possible to establish relationships with a number of companies with potentially conflicting interests.

4.5   INTELLECTUAL PROPERTY

An added dimension to the cost and price issue is the vexed question of ownership of intellectual property. In a true collaboration, all parties are contributing to the collaboration and therefore all should benefit from the results. The problem is that the benefits may be both tangible and intangible, and attributing the value of inputs and outputs involves trying to balance financial and intellectual contributions. It has become a cliché that the output of academic–industrial collaborations is rarely of direct commercial value, but nevertheless it is essential that it should be the case that mechanisms are in place to ensure that such an output is managed and exploited effectively and that all parties receive an appropriate return.

The costs of a project are in principle quantifiable, but the price charged may vary and the main element which is treated as a variable is the overhead component. The main factor, which has been used traditionally in UK universities to determine the level of overhead, is the particular regime adopted for the ownership of intellectual property. In summary, if a company funds a piece of work and insists on ownership of any intellectual property arising with no return to the university share in the benefit, should that intellectual property be successfully commercially exploited, then the university would argue that the project is more like a piece of contract work, and full overheads should be paid. If, however, and this is more common, the work is of genuine mutual interest, a lower overhead might be acceptable. In this case the university would expect to benefit from any commercial success, in the form of a revenue-sharing scheme, although the chances of any real value to the university accruing by this route are recognised as slim, and unlikely to compensate for the trade-off in funding. Under this regime, whether the university or the company owns the intellectual property is to some extent a matter of negotiation, but one which should be driven by a real assessment both of the parties' needs and of obtaining the optimal exploitation strategy for the technology.

Companies frequently argue that exclusive ownership of the intellectual property is crucial to them before they will make a commitment to its exploitation, and certainly this is compounded in the start-up sector by the financiers and venture capitalists, who insist that the companies in which they invest own the technology that they hope to exploit. British Technology Group has always insisted on ownership as a *sine qua non* prior to exploitation. Logically, however, access even on a non-exclusive basis and freedom to exploit are a company's minimum requirement and this can be handled via a licence rather than by an outright assignment. An assignment gives a company the security that it perceives it needs but the difficulty for the university is that it loses control over the technology if the company chooses to sell it on, uses it as a block, or indeed is simply incompetent. Similarly the technology may have applications outside or cease to be part of the core business of the company, in which case again exploitation may not occur.

Conversely companies argue that universities do not have the expertise and resources to defend patents, and only if companies own them will they be prepared to do so. Once again an exclusive licence, whereby these responsibilities are transferred to the company, is an effective way of handling this situation while at the same time protecting the long-term interests of the university.

A further complication is that universities, rightly, will wish to retain the right to use the intellectual property for their own research purposes, and will be reluctant to enter into agreements that limit the scope for collaboration with other companies in the future. Indeed, currently in the UK a part of the funding that universities receive from government is directly proportional to their ability to retain ownership of generic research results arising from collaborative agreements. Paradoxically the pharmaceutical industry, as the major industrial sponsor of academic research, rightly finds these arrangements inappropriate, as it finds it hard to conceive of the situation where it would wish to share the results of the work it has fully funded with a direct competitor through the intermediacy of a university. This is a good example of problems being caused by a global solution being applied to a complex problem.

One of the main frustrations for the academic in an industrial collaboration is the difficulty in publishing. Naturally, in so far as the industrial sponsor sees the results as representative of a commercial advantage, they will wish to see them protected. In some cases, where this involves patent issues, the delay in publishing can be a real disadvantage both to the academic and to their host institution. This conflict is often dealt with by means of a reasonable compromise, which is to allow the company to be informed of the content of publications in advance, and to allow a period of time for it to assess the content for material that needs protecting before publication takes place. Sometimes disagreements occur as to what is a reasonable period, but in practice if the collaboration is proceeding well, and the parties are in good communication with each other, the issue generally resolves itself in practice. Patenting is of vital importance to the pharmaceutical industry, and the filing of a patent initiates a process whereby the preliminary patent is published roughly eighteen months after the first filing. For an academic this is a long delay, but at least there is a default position and clearance for publication can occur much earlier. It is sometimes forgotten that one purpose of patenting is to put information into the public domain, the trade-off being that the individual or company so doing gains the right to prevent other people infringing their position for a period of time. If the aims and objectives of the parties in the collaboration are congruent, they will have a mutual interest in optimising both the protection and publication of results. Generally universities also allow student theses to be examined under conditions of confidentiality and to be kept from public display for reasonable periods to allow protection of results.

More difficult than patents is confidential know-how, as it can be argued that the very status of universities means that all the results of their research should ultimately reach the public domain. If information is generated that is only commercially valuable by virtue of its confidentiality, a problem can arise which can only be dealt with on a case-by-case basis, by close consultation between the parties to reduce as far as possible the amount of material that needs to be kept confidential, and by very careful consideration of the content of publications and theses. In principle, work that is likely to generate such results is best handled by consultancy or by other means than an academic collaboration. It is vital for the success of the collaboration that the issue of publication is dealt with before disputes arise. It is quite possible for the collaborative work to grind to a complete halt in the event of a disagreement and for mistrust to develop.

These factors all need to be taken into account when setting up a collaboration but there are some useful lessons that may be learned from the US and from European collaborations. In the US, in the state universities, research tends to be funded federally, but teaching is funded by the state. In the private sector, teaching is paid for by students' fees and supported by the universities' own endowments whereas research again is largely funded federally. The costs of teaching and research are therefore somewhat easier to disaggregate than in the UK. Overheads are negotiated by each university with the major federal sponsors and applied globally to collaborative projects. Costing and pricing are generally regarded as quite separate issues from the ownership of intellectual property, and indeed in the state sector, state law often requires ownership to remain with the universities and licensing is the norm. Collaborating companies are offered a non-exclusive royalty-free licence to the results of the work they have funded or a first option to a royalty-bearing exclusive licence. This system has the major advantage of establishing a framework for managing intellectual property, and also means that potentially difficult negotiations only occur when there is something worth arguing about.

In Europe, a model collaboration agreement for the Framework programmes has been drafted and the principles are similar. Ownership of intellectual property rests with its generator, all parties in a collaboration have access to the results for their own purposes and if a commercial party exploits the results, an appropriate return will be made to non-commercial parties who do not or can not exploit themselves. Once again a framework has been established and the mechanism is activated only when exploitable intellectual property is generated.

4.6   NEW PATTERNS OF COLLABORATION

These issues, although important and of great consequence to university administrators, are nevertheless tactical and mechanistic rather than strategic, the fundamental issue being the identification of and commitment to realising the mutual benefits that can be obtained from successful links between the two sectors. The scale of that commitment has grown very substantially, and in contrast to the general pattern of links with individual researchers, a large number of very substantial long-term collaborations between single companies and single universities were established in the late 1980s and early 1990s. Notable amongst these was the appearance on the scene of a number of Japanese pharmaceutical companies. Those set up prior to 1986 in the biotechnology sector have been documented in Kenney's book and others in a more recent publication by Webster.[70]

Many of the major universities in the US, e.g. Harvard, MIT, Johns Hopkins, Washington University, have successfully exploited the growing appetite among major companies for collaborative research. At Duke University in North Carolina, a collaborative effort with Glaxo is underway with the group that discovered the relationship between Alzheimer's disease and apolipoprotein E genes. It is now known that individuals with two apoE4 genes develop Alzheimer's disease on average 20 years before those individuals with one apoE2 and one apoE3 gene. Testing for the apoE4 gene has potential to identify susceptibility to Alzheimer's, and supports the diagnosis of a suspected case of the disease—which could be useful in assembling patients for clinical trials for new drugs. The aim of the collaboration is to discover the biochemical mechanism underlying the enhanced risk for Alzheimer's disease, and to develop screens that will permit *in vitro* evaluation of drug candidates that work by this mechanism. The collaboration is very much at the basic end of the research spectrum, but with a clear commercial end-point, and involves molecular biologists at the Glaxo Wellcome Institute for Molecular Biology in Geneva, as well as pharmacologists at Glaxo Wellcome in the UK. As such it seems to satisfy the aims and aspirations of both the academic and industrially minded scientists involved.

Given the developmental timescale of the industry, it is probably too early to assess the real outcomes of these developments but there is no doubt that funding external research may be more cost-effective than employing permanent in-house staff and certainly, given the highly regulated nature of the industry, there exist political pressures on companies to establish R&D activities in the countries where they wish to sell their products. Despite the squeeze on their funding by the Government, universities are reasonably well set up with the basic equipment and facilities needed for research and certainly have the knowledge base from which to grow new projects. If indeed diversity is the key to innovation, and as inventions are rarely generated to order, the value of such links in increasing the likelihood of new breakthroughs is self-evident.

In parallel with these major single company collaborations there have sprung up what have been dubbed by Webster 'Co-locational Collaborations', triggered in part by the availability of space on science parks and in incubator facilities. The nature of these collaborations is somewhat at arm's length, and the benefits indirect rather than direct. They generally consist of a strategic research unit located very close to a major university but initially with no con-tractual relationships, except perhaps relating to payment of rents or the use of university facilities which may include consultancy from individual members of staff. These co-locations seek to maximise the possibility for collaboration, and to provide a university-like environ-ment while retaining normal controls over employees, intellectual property and the nature of the work carried out. Any collaborations that do arise would be put on the normal contractual basis.

In the UK, examples include Smith and Nephew in York, the James Black Foundation (funded by Johnson and Johnson) at King's College London, Sandoz at University College in London, Yamanouchi in Oxford and both Parke Davis and Glaxo Wellcome in Cambridge. The Sandoz and Glaxo Wellcome initiatives are examples of what could be called embedded co-locations in that the company facilities are actually situated within departments of the host universities. These initiatives present a multidisciplinary environment, in medicinal chemistry, biochemistry and pharmacology, for drug discovery. This contrasts with the predilection of university depart-ments to be excellent in core disciplines rather than interactive with complementary ones, and may be an interesting model to watch. One has to ask whether such units have a potential role in collaborating with a number of industrial companies in addition to their main sponsor, and under what circumstances this could happen. The Celltox centre (see p. 160) at the University of Hertfordshire is an example of a small academic unit that serves both academic and industrial sectors, and is in the forefront of alternatives to animal testing for toxicological studies. There are also examples, such as Receptor Research at Exeter University, of small entrepreneurial companies being established in an academic environment; in this case, the company conducts some contractual chemical and biochemical research and can attract industrial partners into the university for other studies with academic investigators. Meanwhile, the typical university facilities, such as the library, present at Exeter offer an excellent environment for a small start-up company. Other drug discovery units with multidisciplinary characteristics have evolved from a university background, such as the UK Strathclyde Institute for Drug Research (SIDR), and the Leiden/Amsterdam Centre for Drug Research (LACDR) in the Netherlands. Both of these are increasingly finding their reputation well served by their track record of scientific endeavour, and the current climate for collaborations between industry and academia. The SIDR has received a total of $8m from industrial sources world-wide to fund development of compounds prior to the stage where they can be licensed out, and is successfully working with Vanguard Medica (q.v.) for development of a psoriasis drug. The LACDR derives half of its income from collaboration from the pharmaceutical industry and other research funding organisations, with the other half from basic university grants. It combines all of the basic disciplines for drug research, from discovery and design to clinical research. For these organisations, their outlook on commercialisation of research places them, and others of their ilk, well for the future.

A further major change in the relationship between companies and universities has resulted from legislative changes in the UK and in the US which have shifted the emphasis from a national system of technology transfer based on a centralised activity to a more fragmented but market-based one located within the universities themselves. In the US, the Bayh–Dole Act of 1980 allowed universities to own and exploit intellectual property arising from publicly funded research.

In the UK, the British Technology Group's monopoly over intellectual property derived from Research Council funded research was removed in 1985. As a result universities were offered the option of exploiting their own inventions, and most chose to do so, setting up technology transfer or technology licensing offices of their own. A few universities chose to remain with BTG which stayed in the public sector until 1995, when it was successfully privatised. It remains one of the world's leading technology transfer organisations within the biomedical sector, a key focus for its business. Universities still form an important source of technology, but increasingly BTG is working with companies themselves to help them exploit their technology.

While the universities generally have acquired the responsibility for exploiting the results of their research work that is funded by the Research Councils, the latter also fund directly a considerable amount of work in their own institutes. In 1990, the Medical Research Council (MRC) set up its own Technology Transfer Group to facilitate links

Cruciform project

The Cruciform project, like Triangle (section 6.7.1.2), grew out of the Glaxo take-over of Wellcome, except this represents the UK rather than the US component. The R&D Director of Wellcome in the UK, Prof. Salvador Moncada, set up the Cruciform project in a disused building which was previously in the University College Hospital in London, together with a number of other Wellcome UK researchers. Currently located at the Rayne laboratories, the first task of the project is to refurbish the old buildings at a cost of £45m before moving in. The project derives its name from the cross-shaped Cruciform building in which it will be housed, and will also be known as the Institute for Strategic Medical Research. Funding is derived from a number of sources, including the Higher Education Funding Council for England (£14.5m), The Wellcome Trust (£11.5m) and Glaxo Wellcome (£10m).

The Cruciform project will sit at the academic–industrial interface, making particular use of contacts in both areas to establish a world centre of excellence in drug discovery research. The project will aim to conduct basic research with a market perspective, away from the direct commercial pressures of industry, in a fertile multidisciplinary academic environment. The primary disciplines involved include medicinal chemistry, basic biology and clinical research. The focus is in the research of cardiovascular disease and neurological disorders such as Alzheimer's disease. The way in which the Cruciform project will operate remains to be seen as time unfolds. At present, the institute can be seen as a provider of focused biomedical research with industrial application, through industrial funds. It is keen not to be seen merely as a provider of contract research, but as a partner to pharmaceutical companies with a meaningful contribution to the thinking processes of research. As such it can provide work to a number of collaborators, for direct funding. Whether the Cruciform project also sees fit to raise money and operate more like a start-up company remains to be seen. Such a move might have the advantage of bringing in more capital.

The Cruciform project has similarities to the William Harvey Institute, also in London, which was set up by the Nobel laureate Sir John Vane in 1986. The primary disciplinary purpose of this institute has been in pharmacology. Like academia, it has become a centre of excellence for research, but it has not been a centre for education, nor has it received substantial public funding. It therefore represents an interesting hybrid, deriving financial support partly from industry, and partly from the medical charities such as The Wellcome Trust. In addition, it has a contract service arm, and runs a number of research conferences, profits from which are used to fund additional research posts.

with industry and to handle the licensing of in-house research to industry. The other Research Councils have generally delegated such activities to their own individual institutions.

Biomedical research in universities is also funded extensively by the major medical charities, which generally hand over the responsibility for exploitation of technology to the universities themselves. These organisations are significant sources of research finance, as mentioned previously (p. 93). Some charities, such as the Cancer Research Campaign (CRC) and the Imperial Cancer Research Foundation, have their own research laboratories and, like the MRC, have their own technology transfer activities. Recently, the Charities Commission has emphasised that charities need to consider the value of their intellectual as well as physical assets. As a result, the charities, notably The Wellcome Trust, are focusing much more explicitly on the exploitation of intellectual property resulting from their funding of research and some commercial ventures (e.g. Cyclacel, from the CRC) have emerged. This is imposing a greater degree of responsibility on the charities and increased complexity in the universities as a result of the latter having to ensure that their responsibilities to their many sponsors are properly discharged. While the increased emphasis on exploiting the output of research is to be welcomed, there is a risk of increasing fragmentation of effort and that an increased administrative burden will reduce the effectiveness with which technology is transferred to industry.

While most basic research does not lead to inventions but leads to results which are disseminated by publication, as a result of these legislative changes the explicit transfer of technology has increased enormously. This has been in the form of the sale and licensing of patents, copyright and other forms of intellectual property to industry and, increasingly, in the creation of new knowledge-based spin-off companies notably in computing, electronics and more recently in the biotechnology sector.

The exploitation of research results by universities is not a simple task as the inventions to be commercialised have arisen not as the result of identified market needs, but often as the by-products of long-term, fundamental research. There is often uncertainty that they will operate outside a laboratory environment and, almost without exception, there is the need for substantial investments of time and money to develop the inventions into products. On the positive side, however, the value of university-derived technology as the feedstock for start-up companies and as a source of new ideas and directions for established companies is now well recognised.

There are a number of salient examples where project-based research has been picked up by industrial sponsors at an early stage, particularly in the area of genomics, which as has been mentioned owes a good deal to its academic provenance. Glaxo Wellcome are collaborating with the Institute of Cancer Research in London on molecular biological approaches to signal transduction, based on the ras-map kinase pathway, which is implicated in abnormal cell differentiation and proliferation, with therapeutic potential in cancer, neurodegeneration and inflammation. SmithKline Beecham are collaborating with RPMS Technology, which is the technology transfer subsidiary of the UK Royal Postgraduate Medical School, to identify potential gene targets in micro-organisms which are involved in pathogenesis. And Roche Bioscience (formerly Syntex) have set up a research alliance with University College London for research into purinoceptors present on neuronal and smooth muscle tissue. All these examples, and many more, have been formed recently because pharmaceutical companies recognise the importance of basic research into diseases, particularly if it can lead to novel biochemical targets which can in turn lead to new and potentially better treatments.

The process by which technology is transferred may be split into several parts: identification of the invention, evaluating whether patent or other forms of protection is appropriate; assessment of the market and determining if additional developmental work is needed; devising an exploitation mechanism whether this be licensing, sales or a company start-up and reducing this to practice; monitoring progress and, if all goes well, collecting revenue and sharing this between the inventors and their university.

Licensing inventions to a company is an effective way of transferring technology and is particularly appropriate in an academic environment as it shifts the financial burden and responsibility from the university to an organisation which, in principle, has greater resources and the diverse skills necessary to take an idea to the market. This leaves the inventors free to carry on with their research, although in some cases, a licence may be accompanied by a consultancy arrangement for the inventors and a further collaboration agreement; thus the overall benefit of the licence to the university may be considerably enhanced. Where additional developmental funds or other resources are needed to take the invention to the proof of principle stage or the technology is generic and capable of multiple applications, formation of a start-up company may be appropriate. Venture capital funding is often required and a considerably higher level of personal commitment from the inventor, although the rewards from an equity share may be substantial. The processes involved from the perspective of the research scientist, and with an emphasis on the biotechnology sector, have been recently described in Sullivan's book on technology transfer.[71]

Conflicts of interest are potentially endemic in all forms of industrial links but no more so than when starting companies. Such conflicts often arise from trying to balance an academic with a business role and may occur as much by accident as by design. Potential abuses include the use of university facilities for personal gain and without compensation to the university, use of publicly funded research workers and students for business purposes, inappropriate attention to university duties (or *vice versa*), shifting research priorities in favour of business, pipelining of inventions to the company and suppression of research findings. The roles of the inventors, the university and their relationships have to be thought through extremely carefully and conflicts of interest managed if not avoided.

Such exploitation is increasingly encouraged by the external pressures on universities to diversify the sources of funding, and to ensure that the maximum dissemination and benefit from the results of their research is realised. Incentive schemes in the form of revenue sharing arrangements for academic inventors have been introduced by the majority of universities, many of whom now have their own companies for the specific purpose of promoting the exploitation of inventions. While this activity is promoting technology transfer it is also leading to fragmentation and competition at perhaps too low a level. The financial returns to the universities, however, will take a long time to accrue as in general university inventions do not result from an explicit market need, are very undeveloped and require an enormous amount of time and money to turn them into a commercial product. Probably only a handful of the large research-based universities have a sufficiently large technology base and critical mass to support self-sustaining technology transfer functions. The US experience, somewhat longer than that of the UK, suggests that a licensing income that exceeds a few percent of the total research budget would be exceptional. This would, nevertheless, amount to very worthwhile sums particularly as the money is unattributed in its use. Turning this argument round, however, the level of investment induced in the economy by the transfer of technology, and by the investment needed to turn these inventions into products, is truly remarkable. The US experience also suggests that the majority of licences are to relatively small companies which do not carry out large amounts of research. Large companies generate their own new leads internally, and have to cope with the problems of internal competition for resources and improving the productivity of their own research.

Every university licensing manager dreams of the blockbuster drug which would bring in massive royalties but the invention of new chemical entities by universities is extremely rare. While the seed corn of drug research is often found in universities, these places do not have the persistence or commercial resources to carry this through to a commercial product. One example where a suite of patents based on a technology rather than a product has produced significant reward is in the Cohen–Baker inventions of 1980, on the principles and tools of genetic engineering. These patents were assigned to Stanford University, who are likely to have received a total of $170m by the time these patents expire in 1997. As regards personal reward, academicians (as opposed to their more financially astute licensing partners) are not generally motivated by monetary gain, which is often achieved by accident. For example, Dr Herschel Smith, while working at the University of Manchester, applied the so-called Birch reduction (named after Professor AJ Birch) to the total synthesis of the novel oral contraceptive norgestrol. This discovery resulted in substantial royalties on the drug sales, and Dr Smith redistributed much of the money he accrued in the form of donations to academic institutions. Another example concerns Professor George Rieveschl, a US academic who discovered the histamine antagonist diphenhy-dramine; at that time royalty income was more modest, and he continued in his career as a research chemist. One of the more recent examples of a drug discovered substantially in academe was atra-curium. This was the brainchild of Professor John Stenlake, and was brought to the market in 1982 as a result of a collaborative effort of the University of Strathclyde and Wellcome Laboratories. It was an improved neuromuscular blocking agent that was used in anaes-thesia. Unlike its forebears, it was not subject to patient variability of liver or kidney metabolic inactivation, but spontaneously lost activity as a result of chemical degradation *in vivo*.

More recently, in the biotechnology sector, the generation of potential therapeutic entities is more common in the academic sector. A considerable number of companies have been spun out of uni-versities to exploit such technology. A number have been set up with the express purpose of garnering technology from a number of universities, and developing these technologies to the point at which they can be licensed on to or jointly developed with a major pharma-ceutical company. This type of company, usually venture capital backed, serves a particularly valuable function in developing academic technology and helping to overcome the problem of critical mass discussed earlier.

Increasingly, academics are seeing opportunities for using their scientific reputations as launching pads for commercial ventures. MacroNex is an example of a company that started life in 1990 with founders from Duke University Medical Center, North Carolina, to discover new treatments for arthritis, atherosclerosis, cancer and AIDS. Ultimately, the company was not successful, as described earlier (p. 87), although other examples of ventures of this kind include

Cantab, a well-established biotechnology company in the UK founded by Dr Alan Munro, the erstwhile acting Head of the Department of Pathology at the University of Cambridge; and Peptide Therapeutics, which was founded by Professor Denis Stanworth from the University of Birmingham. Very close links with the university are maintained, and inventions from academia are progressed in a collaborative way with trust on both sides. As another example of this change in emphasis, some universities now see themselves as organisations with thousands of workers (students and lecturers), led by a Chief Executive who regards his role as commensurate with that of a leader in charge of this size of organisation.

Oxford University has been one of the universities at the forefront of changes in the relationships between industry and academia, and has been heavily involved in the success of Oxford Asymmetry and Oxford Molecular (q.v.). These companies were set up jointly by the university together with Dr Stephen Davies and Professor Graham Richards, respectively, who still retain lectureships at the university in addition to their roles in these small companies. The availability of facilities, such as the excellent nuclear magnetic resonance facilities at the university, is of great help to all new and growing companies that have difficulty in justifying large capital expense early in their life.

4.7   CONCLUSION

Collaboration between the academic sectors and the pharmaceutical industry has been a facet of drug discovery for many years. The place of academia, by its very nature at the frontiers of science, makes it an ideal partner in studies that involve new fields where advances are rapidly occurring. This is different from the role of the CRO, which fits better into defined studies that are necessary for the development of drugs rather than their discovery.

As links between the two sectors increase in scale, scope and strategic content, the lines between the two are becoming increasingly blurred and engendering fears of the loss of impartiality of the public sector research base, and the sequestration of research by the private sector of research funded for the general good. Clear guidelines, proper implementation and identification of what lies within the boundaries of acceptable academic behaviour are required. Flexibility is essential, as the system continues to evolve and changing notions of accountability may be required as a result.[72] Traditional views of the purity of academic research are not based in fact and the long history of linkages between the private and public sectors suggests that these issues can be dealt with and can be actively managed to the mutual advantage of all parties, provided that there is a joint will to succeed, a respect for each other's aims and ambitions, and a sharing in the benefits of success.

5
The Role of CROs and Small Research Companies

5.1 RELATIONSHIP OF CROs TO LARGE PHARMACEUTICAL COMPANIES

5.1.1 Historical perspective

'Contracting out' or to use the more modern idiom, 'outsourcing', has not been a uniformly essential element in the strategy of pharmaceutical companies. Although outsourcing chemical scale-up and, more particularly, bulk manufacturing has always been an integral part of the activities of the pharmaceutical industry, outsourcing of biology has been a more recent phenomenon. The reason for this is that the more mature industrial chemical industry was already using contract providers, and this service became available for the younger pharmaceutical industry. Chemical plant is expensive and to maintain profitability it needs to be fully utilised. The use of such equipment for a number of clients has obvious cost-saving elements. There was neither the requirement nor the services available for there to be a need to consider outsourcing biological studies. However, one single event in 1955, namely the tragedy of thalidomide, transformed this situation and this was followed later by another event in 1975, the introduction of Good Laboratory Practice (GLP). Since these two events, the industry has accepted that outsourcing preclinical safety studies has been an integral and essential part of their overall strategy. Similar comments apply to the clinical work that is performed to supply proof of safety and efficacy of new medicines, although this remains outside the ambit of this book.

Two basic reasons underlie this situation. One is a reality and the second, arguably, a perception. The reality was that the industry was on a very steep upward drug discovery curve. It was just not physically possible for companies to build toxicology facilities fast enough to cope with the plethora of compounds emerging from the golden era of drug discovery. There was also, even in those heady days, the recognition of the high level of risk associated with drug discovery and development and a strategy to resource internally to the level of the troughs and to outsource the peaks. Of course there had to be service providers to meet this strategy and it is interesting in the context of today's talk of preferred providers, strategic alliances and partnerships that Beecham Research Laboratories in 1966 agreed to an alliance and preferred provider relationship with the newly formed Huntingdon Research Centre (HRC) laboratories to help ensure the latter's financial stability and long-term future as a CRO.

The second reason for the growth of the biological contract research business was the 'independence' of CROs undertaking safety studies. The commercial integrity of the pharmaceutical industry has always been perceived as suspect and this was extended to its technical performance when fraudulent activity was exposed by the FDA. With this background and the box-ticking regulatory-driven bureaucratic mentality of government agencies, the industry became convinced that preclinical safety studies, especially the long-term 'feed and bleed' toxicology studies, were best handled by CROs. These studies were an essential part of their core business of marketing new products but they sat very uncomfortably in an industry that, to be successful, had to generate an atmosphere of creativity and innovation. There was a perception that the routine, large-scale requirements that were increasingly imposed upon the industry by regulation in the late 1960s, 1970s and 1980s were best handled by external contractors who specialised in attention to detail rather than leaps of thought.

5.1.2   The needs of the industry in the 1970s and 1980s

Such was the dependence of the industry on CROs during this time, it would be overstating the position of the CROs to be called a service industry. Just as the industry itself saw a very short healthcare chain (obtaining a product licence), so the CRO industry had little concept of a customer. Despite the rapid growth and number of CROs, there was business enough for all. The pharmaceutical industry itself could not develop their compounds fast enough and there was no time to discuss or argue internally or externally with the regulatory authorities whether a study should or should not be done. The *modus operandum* was to book a slot at a CRO and tick the regulatory box.

The regulatory drive was exacerbated by the variations of guidelines not only within Europe but particularly between Japan, Europe and the US. This very often meant performing additional studies providing little or no added value in terms of safety information, and sometimes studies were duplicated, with the obvious inherent dangers of apparently new findings arising from biological variation. On more than one occasion has a company fallen foul of the strategy of simply repeating a study for completion of a local registration. Since it is incumbent upon sponsors to submit all preclinical safety data to every regulatory authority this can cause considerable concern and ensuing delays. This was a situation of more haste less speed.

The approach taken by companies in response to regulatory demands has been examined by reviewing the toxicology data submitted to the UK registration authorities for three injectable β-lactam antibiotics, methicillin, ticarcillin and temocillin.[73] The amount of data submitted for methicillin in 1960 was contained in 10 pages which were published in the open scientific literature. This contrasts with 2500 pages for temocillin which was registered in 1984 and the data for which were unpublished. Considering the acute life-threatening bacterial infections all these antibiotics were treating, the value added by the large preclinical toxicology package for temocillin in terms of clinical safety was very small.

In this climate there was little need for CROs to undertake any significant business development activities. There was an excess of demand over supply that meant that sponsors had to book slots well in advance, and CROs could easily fill spaces due to cancellations with alternative studies.

The studies were characterised by being predominantly subchronic or chronic toxicology studies, carcinogenicity studies and reproductive toxicology studies. These studies, though long, were easily scheduled and with bleeds and necropsies determined and upfront by protocol, they were easily planned. With good organisation through study directors and attention to GLP at the operational level, scientific input was minimal. Typically, if there were no problems, sponsors would visit periodically to satisfy regulatory requirements and very regrettably, and irresponsibly too, sponsors gave the CRO little or no information on the compound they were handling and studying. The phenomenon of staff in CROs knowing only the colour and code number of the compound was not an unusual one. This was done in the name of secrecy. This mentality arose from the fear that a competitor also using the same CRO might stumble upon some useful information during a visit, or worse still the CRO might be less than honest and share the information with a competitor. The message generally from sponsors was that the CRO should perform the study exactly as written in the protocol and report the findings, since only the sponsor should interpret the results.

Relationships of servant (service) master (customer) developed. This progressed for some into loyal and lasting professional relationships, but for most it was one based on business expediency with little or no recognition of true mutual professional respect. The Japanese pharmaceutical industry, even younger than that in the US and Europe, was among those that developed loyal ties. They were understandably very concerned to learn quickly and catch up. Together with the Japanese culture for business loyalty, this produced very strong scientific and professional relationships if not business alliances.

From the CRO perspective there was little or no risk and indeed the sponsor was not asking the CRO to accept any risk. This was in fact part of the great culture divide that separated the two otherwise mutually dependent partners. The Western sponsor would normally spread his outsourcing risk by working with several CROs. Putting all your eggs in one basket in a new and rapidly expanding industry seemed to make little scientific or commercial sense. This was not a problem to the CRO either. There was relatively little risk of compounds in long-term toxicology and carcinogenicity studies not going to completion and CROs were more than happy to have the widest possible base of financially sound large companies as clients. It was also true that CROs developed selective expertise and came to offer 'niche' services, e.g. genetic toxicology testing. As a result, sponsors were able to choose particular CROs, not so much on the basis of price, but on expertise and experience.

The 1970s and early 1980s were golden years for both the product-based and the service industry. As a whole each was dependent on the other. Then having established its tremendous industrial business strength, the pharmaceutical industry decided that it would invest heavily in building pharmaceutical development facilities so that it need not be dependent on others. Dependency on CROs was seen as a sign of vulnerability. The future was in more new products, some of which promised to be blockbusters, and developing these valuable products was seen as better performed by the experienced and integrated in-house personnel. CROs were a second-best option, having no real business, personal or professional equity in these complex molecules. So in the mid- to late 1980s many of the major pharmaceutical companies built or purchased extensive preclinical safety evaluation facilities. Some of these companies still proposed operating as in the past on the strategy of using CROs for peak demand, but the overall strategy was to be involved with CROs less than before. Of course, this assumed that the overall business would continue as before. In the event, as we now know, it did not. It says something of an industry which claims premiership in technical and business innovation that it did not see the new but dark dawn until it had burdened itself with preclinical development facilities and staff of enormous proportions. One can only speculate at the number of rodent and canine buildings with all the infrastructure of plant, clean and dirty corridors, stand-by generators and so on that were built in the mid to late 1980s. It led to an enormous capacity in the industry as a whole.

5.1.3   The needs of the industry in the 1990s and beyond

The various pressures placed upon the pharmaceutical industry in the late 1980s and 1990s are outlined in the Introduction and will not be repeated here. As discussed, the impact on R&D has been very substantial, and in turn the impact on those industries providing services to R&D such as CROs has been very profound.

Two major factors, one negative and one positive, are operating to affect the dynamics of the CRO business. The negative factor is the consolidation by either acquisition or merger of the big and medium-sized pharmaceutical companies. The increased capacity for internal discovery and development generated by these companies, as mentioned earlier, contributes to this negative situation. The positive factor is the increasing hunger of the industry for excellent development candidates, and that candidates emanating from extramural institutions are an option that must be pursued.

Within these two major opposing factors are other factors which influence the direction of the equation. On the negative side it is quite clear that the industry cannot afford to fund large Phase III clinical trials on multiple compounds. Selection criteria for compounds entering development need to be strictly adhered to, and even if accepted following critical review of the science and commercial potential, may suffer in the overall prioritisation process when compounds are compared. As has been discussed earlier in this book, there is unlikely to be a shortage of new leads and development candidates for selection and exploratory development, but there needs to be a much improved filtering system that only allows the few high-priority compounds into the later and vastly more expensive stages of development. Thus the traditional bread-and-butter long-term toxicology, carcinogenicity and reproductive toxicology studies on which the CRO industry was originally based will decline. But the negative impact does not end there. Since international harmonisation of preclinical safety guidelines there has already been a reduction in the length of chronic rodent toxicology testing (12 months to 6 months) and it seems probable that over time we shall see a further curtailment of chronic toxicology testing (12 months to 9 or 6 months in the dog) and in carcinogenicity testing in rodents. New models such as transgenic animals when introduced and validated may also have an impact on the reduction in chronic animal studies. Furthermore, the attitudes of regulatory authorities and pharmaceutical companies have changed since the 1970s and 1980s. Greater flexibility on behalf of these agencies and the recognition that good science makes good regulatory sense has thrown the onus back to the scientist to justify on a case-by-case basis the preclinical safety programme. These arguments need to cover why certain studies might be omitted without compromising overall clinical safety assessment for the particular therapeutic condition being pursued.

Rational, rather than ritualistic, preclinical development is now the order of the day. There remain strong regulatory factors to be considered in determining developmental work, particularly as the harmonisation across national authorities has in some senses increased rigidity, but there has also been an increased recognition of science as a driving force behind the regulatory process in the 1990s. This is highlighted by consideration of the new therapeutic agents coming from the advances in biotechnology such as recombinant therapeutic proteins and gene therapies. These biotechnological compounds cannot be considered by the same testing paradigms as traditional low-molecular-weight new chemical entities. The studies have to be designed and tailored to the specific activity and general chemical and biological properties of the compound. In general with these products, it will be scientifically inappropriate to conduct chronic safety studies in animals. The International Conference on Harmonisation (ICH) has discussed what guidance to give applicants in this rapidly growing area of biologicals and biopharmaceuticals. It is clear from these that a generalised prescriptive set of studies has yet to be produced—in fact it may not be possible to produce. In its place are guidance notes for the applicant to consider what might be the most appropriate type of studies to be performed.

Overall preclinical safety assessment is now focusing on the very early stages of exploratory development to support Phase I and II clinical studies, and a more flexible and scientific approach to preclinical safety programmes is being adopted. This of course presents a completely different picture from the situation of the previous decades, and for the traditional CRO who wishes to be involved in such studies, a completely different approach to servicing their large

pharmaceutical clients is required. This phase of compound development has been seen by such sponsor companies as well within the
domain of their internal expertise, for which extensive facilities exist,
which need to be used—as far as possible—to capacity. They have felt
these early critical phases would be best entrusted to their
enlightened and highly committed internal staff. However, it is
inevitable that as CROs change their culture and adapt to the new
environment and as further pressure on the R&D budget is applied,
as it surely will, that these large companies will outsource these
earlier phases of the development process. Indeed the combination
of the traditional lean and hungry CRO together with the newly
acquired culture of scientific flexibility makes for a formidable
development force in terms of costs and speed of development. The
internal bureaucracies and financial overheads of large pharmaceutical companies are unlikely to be able to match these standards of
time and costs.

The number of CROs in Europe and North America has continued
to increase in the 1990s, although at a slower rate than in the 1970s
and 1980s. There are about 800 such organisations world-wide, about
half of these in Europe. A small minority of these organisations have
gone out of business since 1993, and about an equal number have
merged or changed ownership. The service-minded culture of these
companies means that disruption to clients is minimised when
mergers and acquisitions occur. Only a small proportion are publicly
traded companies, whose share prices have increased markedly in
recent times; the vast majority of CROs are, however, privately held.
The bulk of growth in the past few years in the industry has been in
the large CROs, who have expanded their range of services. Particular
areas of growth have been in quality assurance, and in conducting
large multicentre international clinical trials, for which the large CROs
are well suited. The turnover of the 12 major companies has been
estimated at $1.2bn in 1995. The total for the sector as a whole in
Europe and North America was $3.5bn for the same period, although
the private ownership of most of the companies involved makes this
a difficult figure to estimate.[52] The current proportion of pharmaceutical R&D which is conducted by CROs is estimated to be around
15–20%, although this proportion varies from company to company.
Recently, it has been reported that around 25% of Glaxo Wellcome's
R&D budget is spent outside the company, with the proportion in
toxicology as high as 50%. The trend for greater outsourcing has led
US analysts to predict growth rates within the CRO industry to be in
the range of 20–25% up until the year 2000. The greatest potential
area for future growth by CROs is into earlier development and

research. Involvement in this area of work is also being viewed by some CROs as a way of attracting customers at an earlier stage of development, with obvious opportunities to retain them during later phases too.

If the large companies are reluctant, at least for the moment, to outsource some of their early selection and exploratory development activities, the small emerging pharmaceutical companies have no option but to use CROs to develop their ideas and products emanating therefrom. Typically these companies are dependent on venture capital funding to develop their innovative technology to commercial success, but have no or little development expertise with which to achieve this. Furthermore, as was mentioned in section 2.8, because the burn rate in pharmaceutical biotechnology is generally very high, speed of development is essential. In addition, if a public flotation and/or licensing to a major company is envisaged then early studies in man to demonstrate proof of principle or other defined clinical milestones are very important in adding value to the asset.

Recognising this opportunity, Corning Pharmaceutical Services (now Covance) launched a campaign in 1992/3 in the US and Europe to assist small companies to achieve rapid development of their innovations. Through a very close consultative and technical partnership between the scientists in both companies, very impressive results have been achieved in Europe by 'fast-tracking' compounds through preclinical development to Phase I and in some cases to Phase II and Phase III. Typically, although this is naturally compound specific, entry into Phase I volunteers can be achieved in 4–6 months and in Phase II studies in patients within 9 months from receipt of compound.[74] Quintiles have more recently also established a dedicated unit to help emerging companies.

The added value to the small company when such studies are successful can be enormous. It is recognised that the risk to investors in such companies is very high and this factor is built into venture capital funding in terms of appropriate rewards to investors. But what of the CRO who has made a very large contribution to the added value? The CRO's input is not limited to having conducted the studies in a GLP-compliant environment; the CRO has also provided considerable personal expertise as well as organisational and operational commitment to achieving the timelines. Typically, in the past there has been no recognition of the subsequent success (or failure) of products developed by CROs. The basis of this situation was that the pharmaceutical company carried all of the risk and the CRO none. However, in the new environment of the 1990s perhaps this situation should be reviewed.

The position today is that CROs carry more risk than in the 1970s and 1980s, as a result of working more flexibly, and in the earlier phases of selection and drug development. Delays due to problems with compound synthesis and pharmaceutical studies can and often do lead to delays in agreed start-up dates. Even worse, scheduled programmes all the way through to Phase I can suddenly and without warning be aborted, through compound-related problems or financial problems of the company. At the same time the CRO is adding value in providing scientific experience, expertise and project management. In these circumstances it may be reasonable to consider that some of the added value is realised by the CRO as well as by the client.

If the relationship between service provider and customer is going to change beyond that expressed above and along the lines suggested in section 3.4 then there certainly does have to be a change in business practice. Proactively introducing new technologies and biological models requires a considerable investment in people, facilities and time. It carries risks well beyond those traditionally accepted by CROs, and needs to be covered financially. Such studies should not require a learning process by the CRO that slows the development of new compounds. A good example in the toxicology area is the development and validation of new *in vitro* technologies that might replace *in vivo* models, and which will satisfy regulatory authorities and scientific peer review. There has been a huge amount of effort and investment into finding alternatives to the notorious *in vivo* Draize eye irritation test in rabbits; it is very sobering indeed that despite these efforts, it has been concluded that none of the nine *in vitro* tests studied met any of the four performance targets set for the validation study.[75] CROs who invested resources into this area on the basis that there would be scientific and regulatory acceptance of the methods must be hugely disappointed from a business as well as a scientific and ethical point of view. One might ask what effect this experience will have on future investment in this area? Unless the industry is prepared to contribute through reasonable profit margins to the innovation drive within CROs they will understandably be somewhat reticent in investing in new technologies.

Unfortunately the trend has been just the other way. With the pressures on the R&D budgets, cutting costs has been the focus. Professional purchasing managers have been brought into the process of negotiating and agreeing the increasing outsourcing activities to drive down fixed internal overheads. The number of CROs with which a single company works has been reduced from as many as

40–50 down to as few as 3–5 for 75% of their outsourced development work. The principle behind these changes has been to save costs, with less attention to quality. Such an attitude may be appropriate for the more manual and physical jobs such as contract cleaning, security, catering and maintenance services, but extending this to scientific services is much more questionable. The principle might be correct but the manner and approach taken to negotiations and discussions has to be fundamentally different. Often this is not the case. For instance one large pharmaceutical company operates a tendering system with CROs as one might expect from an architect obtaining quotes from building contractors for a project. Whilst the company might say that they also take into account the unquantifiable added value of experience and expertise when considering the tenders, it hardly fulfils the criteria for an open and flourishing business partnership, let alone one in which the scientists need to work very closely to deliver good quality science and a timely report.

There is no question that such practices have led to preclinical CRO work being financially undervalued. As a result some CROs are working on very low or no profit margin just to remain in business. The preclinical CRO organisations are thus in danger of being seen as a commodity business that can be screwed down on the basis of the economic theory of supply and demand. This approach is to fundamentally misunderstand the strategic importance of the CRO in the pharmaceutical industry's core business of producing innovative therapies. It is essential that the pharmaceutical industry does not continue down this path and recognises that it is dependent on a financially buoyant, flourishing and innovative CRO industry. The point has been raised earlier as to whether there is already sufficient choice of service providers from which the industry can choose. The changes in the marketplace mentioned above, whether they be deliberate or unintentional, will do nothing to increase diversity and choice for the customer.

How has the CRO industry responded to this new environment? Like the industry it serves, there has been consolidation. In the UK two of the major preclinical CROs have recently merged (Huntingdon Research Centre (HRC) and Life Science Research (LSR) to form HLS—Huntingdon Life Sciences). Toxicol Laboratories have been acquired by Quintiles. Although there is still room for niche CROs the trend has been to provide a wide range of pharmaceutical development services in one organisation. The largest of these CROs is Covance which has a staff of over 3500 and covers preclinical, clinical, clinical laboratory testing, clinical trials packaging and biologicals manufacture. As in any large international organisation, integrating its own activities presents internal problems, but the real business challenge is to use this very large development resource to optimise the drug development process for the benefit of the pharmaceutical industry. The CRO business is highly competitive and in this respect it is similar to the product-based industry it serves. However, there is a major difference in the way the two industries compete for business. The pharmaceutical industry can hope to differentiate very clearly its products based on hard data obtained from efficacy, safety and pharmacoeconomic studies. Even in today's new healthcare environment, the marketplace is poorly sensitive to price when clear product advantage can be shown. In addition, the international marketplace provides a huge customer base. This is in marked contrast to the CRO industry which has an ever shrinking number of large well-founded mature customers and a large number of young, small and venture-capital-hungry customers. Differentiating and selling technical services to a highly intelligent R&D management is far removed from marketing products to doctors and healthcare providers. Like the situation of purchasing managers negotiating prices with suppliers and providers the principles might be the same but the attitudes and approaches need to be quite different.

Simply telling customers that studies can be completed faster, error-free and reported to agreed timelines is not always credible. Their initial reaction is to believe that all CROs make these same claims; and to ask what is the real added value that an individual CRO might uniquely offer. Given that the facilities, GLP status and technical competence and the like are undifferentiated for the successful CRO, the simple answer has to be knowledge and experience. This is perhaps exemplified by the fact that Corning-Besselaar was involved with the progression of six NDAs in 1994, and five in 1993, a level of experience that very few large pharmaceutical companies (let alone small ones) can match. Specific technologies might for a short time provide uniqueness, e.g. inhalation technology, continuous infusion technology, telemetry, transgenics, etc., but enduring added value can only come from a strong knowledge base of the core business. In this case this is the technical and scientific complexity of the pharmaceutical development process. CROs who can capture this knowledge through employing professionally experienced leaders, who can then cultivate the scientific culture of pharmaceutical development into their organisation, will be the winners of the fight to capture increased market share in a generally mature or shrinking market.

5.2 PRACTICE

5.2.1 Chemistry

The outsourcing of chemistry has been a routine operation for many of the later-stage manufacturing operations relating to bulk production. The techniques, plant, operating conditions and expertise that may apply to specific transformations lend themselves ideally to contractual operation. By comparison, laboratory scale chemistry and the procedures required for synthesis of research quantities of material are sufficiently flexible to be done very efficiently in the multipurpose environment of an in-house medicinal chemistry group, where interaction with the biologist can be maximised.

Despite these comments, there are various niche areas in which contract chemistry has gained a foothold, particularly combinatorial chemistry (see section 5.2.1.2).

5.2.1.1 Discovery chemistry

For the reasons given above, it is rare to find discovery chemistry conducted by contract (except as part of a multidisciplinary project—see section 5.3). There are a number of difficulties associated with this practice.

Foremost among these is the fact that the inventiveness that underpins successful medicinal chemistry is difficult to dissociate from the practice of that research. The provision of ideas is inseparable from discovery chemistry, and a major part of the motivation for the people who do it. It is difficult to foresee discovery chemistry being routinely best done by contract unless the contractor has an intellectual stake in the project. Such a stake would normally require some ownership of intellectual property shared with the client partner. Few contract discovery companies have been able to establish relationships with major partners except in areas of niche expertise. By and large, medicinal chemistry is conducted efficiently, flexibly and to a high standard in large pharmaceutical companies. The opportunities for contract discovery chemistry have not developed sufficiently to allow a diverse, quality industry to grow.

It has been possible to set up core units in other than purely industrial settings, such as the academic institutes described in chapter 4. These units have not served as contractual discovery chemistry groups. Indeed their strategic purpose has at times seemed confused. Nevertheless, these ventures have been preferred in the past to setting up contractual arrangements of the type routinely conducted in more biological sciences.

In addition to the issue of ownership of intellectual property, three other factors have contributed to the difficulty of contracting discovery medicinal chemistry. One is need for iteration in the discovery process, necessitating close interaction between chemist and biologist (see section 1.2.4). Second is the advantage of interaction between chemists working in different areas, whose common expertise could, if kept together, offer synergies to each other's work. Because many of the techniques in medicinal and synthetic organic chemistry have commonality whatever the therapeutic target, there is much to be said for cross-fertilisation in this discipline across project groups (by comparison, such cross-fertilisation may be less advantageous in pharmacology). Third, the fact that a large contract discovery chemistry sector has not developed has led to concerns that what does exist is of poorer quality than can be found in larger pharmaceutical companies although in niche areas this precept is currently being challenged.

As a result of these factors, contract discovery chemistry is comparatively rare. Contractors are often used, however, for resynthesis of compounds for more detailed pharmacological profiling. Such work is often needed when initial screening of a compound yields results that warrant more extensive investigation in a number of animal models. However, the difficulty of arranging this work to be done suggests that it should be done on a regular, rather than one-off, basis and for a number of compounds of related synthetic provenance rather than individual in their synthetic route. For instance, Chiroscience have used a group of Polish chemists for such a purpose, and there are other groups of talented chemists from the former Eastern bloc and the ex-USSR for which there may be some financial advantage due to a lower cost base.

Some of the contractors offering contract discovery chemistry in the UK and US are shown in Table 5.1. In addition to these contract-based arrangements, various strategic alliances have evolved between small emerging companies as providers of discovery chemistry for larger partners. Examples include Oxford GlycoSystems and Upjohn, and Glycomed (now Ligand) with Sankyo. Both of these projects are in the area of adhesion inhibitors.

5.2.1.2   *Combinatorial chemistry*

A particularly popular area where specialist technology is being offered by contract or in a collaborative setting is combinatorial

Table 5.1　Discovery chemistry and laboratory-scale custom synthesis providers

Name	Location	Country
Albany Molecular Research	Albany, NY	US
ChemBiochem Research	Utah	US
Organix	Woburn, MA	US
Regis Technologies Inc	Morton Grove, IL	US
Synthetech	Albany, OR	US
Aston Molecules[a]	Birmingham	UK
Tocris Cookson Chemicals	Southampton	UK
Key Organics	Cornwall	UK
Macfarlan Smith	Edinburgh	UK
Maybridge	Cornwall	UK
Merlin	Wye	UK
Ultrafine	Salford	UK
SPECS	The Hague	Netherlands

[a] Recently purchased by Oncogene Sciences.

chemistry (see section 1.2.2).[76] The partnerships that have been formed go beyond a contract setting. Collaborations of varying kinds have been developed, including strategic alliances and even mergers and acquisitions (see later). For this section, and later on when automated methods, high-throughput screening and molecular biology are discussed, the notion of a CRO needs to be enlarged to encompass small biotechnology companies as providers. Such companies exist for other purposes than merely to service clients, as a CRO generally does. They often have their own proprietary research interests, and may even cling to a desire to carry one of their inventions through to the market in the absence of any collaborative arrangements.

The president of one combinatorial chemistry company, Combi-Chem, predicted in 1994 that 'every company doing small molecule drug discovery has to have access to combinatorial chemistry, or they won't be competitive 5 years from now'. Such sentiments are widely held at senior positions within large pharmaceutical companies too, and place providers of combinatorial chemistry expertise in a powerful position.[76] In an effort to make good use of this technology, large pharmaceutical companies and small combinatorial chemistry providers have forged partnerships in three ways:

- strategic alliances
- flexible contracts
- acquisition (partial or complete)

Examples of the latter include Glaxo's purchase of Affymax for $533m in March 1995. Affymax have focused their efforts on the synthesis of peptides and antibodies as well as other small molecules. Amongst a broad portfolio, they have a method for encoding the structure of the synthesised compound by using a tagging technique for each microscopic bead that the compound is synthesised upon. Affymax have said that exploitation of their technologies has benefited greatly from the take-over by Glaxo. Full integration with a very large pharmaceutical partner is seen by Affymax as preferable to the rather looser arrangement that previously existed within various partnerships with a number of companies. Acquisition is also the route that has been followed by Selectide (purchased by Marion Merrell Dow (now Hoechst Marion Roussel) in January 1995), and Sphinx Pharmaceuticals (acquired by Lilly in September 1994). These earlier takeovers may have contributed to Glaxo's decision to acquire Affymax, in so far as they created a climate in which large companies with a commitment to this technology saw the availability of small company partners diminishing. Whether Glaxo were right to pay such a large sum for Affymax is not yet assessable. However, having fixed their relationship in this way, they were assured that a competitor could not impede their continuing desire to work with Affymax.

The purchase of Selectide by Hoechst Marion Roussel has been stated to comply with the latter's strategy to enhance the flow of commercially attractive products emanating from R&D. As evidence of the power of combinatorial chemistry for generation of lead compounds, Selectide have identified SEL 2906 as a product for anti-coagulation/anti-thrombosis, for which filing of an IND is planned. The basis of the purchase of Sphinx Pharmaceuticals by Lilly is likewise attributed to strengthening the capability to turn lead compounds into therapies.

An example of a slightly less rigid integration is to be found in the relationship of Chiron and Ciba (now Novartis). In 1994, Ciba acquired a minority 49% of Chiron, and the latter acquired a diagnostics division of Ciba, together with a joint venture between the two companies on vaccines called Biocine. Despite the close ties between the two companies, Ciba has permitted Chiron the freedom to involve itself with other partners based around its core combinatorial technology, such as with KOSAN Biosciences and Japan Tobacco. This clearly has advantages for Chiron, but does it help Ciba? One libertarian view would suggest that by having to compete with other combinatorial companies in the partnership 'market', Chiron need to maintain their technological lead. (Chiron are one of the more established companies in this area, and their credibility is high.) Ciba benefit from such a partner, who is technologically advanced, well respected, and is receptive to the changing demands placed upon it by potential partners who are still learning how best to use this technology for the ends of drug research.

As an alternative to complete or partial acquisition, many large companies have formed alliances or long-term contracts with combinatorial chemistry partners. These alliances are popular means for developing expertise in this area, and are typically based on the following components:

- Upfront fee (in return for exclusivity in a particular area)
- Equity investment
- Funding of activity based on 'full-time equivalents' (FTEs) and a specified number of years of commitment
- Milestone payments (such as when a lead is defined, when a compound enters development and when clinical trials are started)
- Royalties (based on a certain percentage of eventual sales, around 5–10%)

The figure associated with the overall deal is calculated with all of these components included, and can give rise to the numbers of $10–50m typically quoted. However, it is clearly evident that the actual monetary transactions that take place will usually not meet this upper limit unless the collaboration results in a marketed compound. It is nevertheless common practice to use this limit as a guide to the size of the deal, and very much in the interests of the smaller partner as it offers reassurance to the investment community as to its financial viability. These comments and remarks on deal structure have applicability to biotechnology company partnerships in other areas, such as in genomics and screening methods (see sections 5.2.2 and 5.2.3.1). A recent review of each of these components in a number of deals has concluded that the average total payments to technology providers of combinatorial chemistry, genomics or gene therapy amounted to $37.4m.[28] Contributions to R&D expenditure and milestone payments are the greatest of these components.

A summary of some of the major initiatives in combinatorial chemistry is shown in Table 5.2, along with other forms of partnership between combinatorial chemistry providers and large pharmaceutical companies. In addition to areas of work covered under these strategic alliances, these small companies also often have other research projects of their own directed towards specific biological targets. Strategic alliances with one partner do not rule out other forms of collaboration with other partners. Combinatorial chemistry companies often engage in a number of contracts or alliances, offering their specialist expertise widely. It is now possible to enter into arrangements with companies merely on the basis of the provision of libraries of compounds for screening, such as Panlabs/Tripos with their venture Optiverse. The library is to contain 100 000 compounds, designed with a highly diverse range of structures in mind. The commercial arrangements are based on a typical contractor/service approach which sets this provider apart from most of the other small combinatorial companies. Panlabs is also able to screen compounds in a number of traditional receptor binding or enzyme bioassays. The incorporation of Tripos into the frame offers the potential for QSAR analysis of active structures. This option has recently been used by Karo Bio in a programme to search for compounds that interact with cell nucleus receptors.

Most of the current activity in combinatorial chemistry is evident in the USA. This is an observation common to other small providers of pharmaceutical technology, and is worthy of some comment. The reorganisations of large pharmaceutical companies began earlier in the US than in other countries in the wake of the election of President Clinton; associated with these changes were rationalisations that spawned many start-up research ventures. There were prominent management theorists in the US such as Stephen Roach, Chief Economist at Morgan Stanley, arguing for rationalisation and corporate downsizing as a method of improving productivity, and in that ensuing process, many highly qualified people were lost from the large pharmaceutical companies. The availability of venture capital is another very major factor; others undoubtedly include the conduciveness of the US tax, legal and bureaucratic systems to business, and the particular strength of the entrepreneurial spirit in the US. By comparison, these changes in the industry at large have hit other countries relatively later on. Thus the UK only features once or twice in Table 5.2, with Oxford Diversity and Peptide Therapeutics, although there are other combinatorial chemistry programmes in place such as the research collaboration of Zeneca pharmaceuticals with Drs Chris Abell and Shankar Balasubramanian at Cambridge University.

In this light, Pfizer's decision to use Oxford Diversity in the UK as its partner for assistance in development of a combinatorial programme is interesting. Prior to the establishment of the alliance, Oxford Diversity had no track record in combinatorial chemistry.[77] Pfizer have stated their choice-reflected faith in Oxford Diversity's entrepreneurial approach and broad expertise in a variety of synthetic methods. They felt they could count on Oxford Diversity to develop a broad range of combinatorial techniques through its talented, young and motivated people. These reasons hark back to some of the issues raised in chapter 2.

Continental European start-up companies in combinatorial chemistry are still embryonic in nature. Even including the UK, Europe is substantially weaker than the US in its biotechnology sector. In terms of pure statistics, the number of firms in Europe in 1995 represented about 40% of those in the US (584 firms vs 1308).[78] However, in terms of R&D spending and numbers of people employed, the proportions are much lower, about 10–15% respectively; much of the European activity is concentrated in the UK, which represents the major site for biotechnological investment, more than matching that in France and Germany combined. In combinatorial chemistry in particular, as well as other areas in which there are weaknesses, European companies are making use of the expertise in the US rather than seeking local providers. (A survey by the Institute of Biotechnology of US biotechnology companies in 1995 showed that 25% of research alliances involved a European partner, with that proportion increasing in 1996.) Despite the strength of the German chemical industry, combinatorial chemistry is only weakly represented in Germany at this stage, with examples such as that of Jerini Biotools in Berlin; in Denmark, there is only AudA pharmaceuticals, which specialises in analogues built around natural product templates. However, it is interesting to note that the three major Swiss companies have been active in a number of venture capital funds with interests in a variety of biotechnology companies. The recent merger of Ciba and Sandoz to form Novartis has been accompanied by the provision of a fund of SFr100m to support new biotechnology companies that may arise in Basle from the rationalisation that will follow the merger. With the exception of the formation of an affiliate to CytoTherapeutics (Modex) in Lausanne, so far there have been very few start-up companies in Switzerland itself, either in combinatorial chemistry or in other areas such as genomics.

California has been a highly favoured location for biotechnology providers in general, and combinatorial chemistry is no exception. One factor, which it enjoys in common with other sites such as Boston in the US and Cambridge or Oxford in the UK, is access to a major research university (Berkeley). However, California is bigger than these examples in terms of the size and success of its biotechnology sector. There is much in the culture of this part of the USA which engenders entrepreneurialism, and much recent history of its success in both the biomedical and computer sectors. Not only are the most established, larger biotechnology companies such an Amgen and Genentech located here, but in the computing industry, the area around San Francisco known as Silicon Valley is synonymous with high-growth, high-risk ventures. By comparison, the European experience is small scale. The most determined effort to create a similar environment in Europe is in France, at Sophia-Antipolis. Like Silicon Valley, this development is located in a beautiful area, with access to sun, sea, mountains and the culture of the Côte d'Azur. There is much to attract the geographically mobile scientist to this location, and the French government has invested over FF1500m (approx. £200m) in making it work. However, despite some success in certain areas of high technology, pharmaceuticals represent only 5% of the employment in the area. The companies represented have yet to establish themselves in terms of partnerships with many of the larger multinationals. Sophia-Antipolis is hardly a failure in terms of technological process, but in bioscience it has lacked the zest of many of the US enterprises. The frontier spirit, the do-or-die instinct, is perhaps easier to find in a population of immigrants who went there to build the West of America, and who are familiar with risk from their beginnings with the highs and lows of the gold rush.

5.2.1.3   Development chemistry

As explained earlier (see section 1.3), the chemical development of a new drug substance involves more than merely reproducing the synthesis on a larger scale to afford quantities of material for toxicology and clinical trials. The key additional elements include process development and analytical support. The latter are occasionally offered by the chemical development provider, although they may otherwise readily be obtained from a large number of analytical support laboratories (which are listed in the back of trade journals such as *Chemistry in Britain* and *Chemical & Engineering News* or can be identified from registers from Technomark[52] or from Soteros[53]).

However, there is a general weakness among many collaborators in regard to chemical process development. This is a vital component of successful chemical development, as has been stressed before (see section 1.3). Without it, a CRO may complement the pilot-plant operations of the in-house chemical development team, but can be of little help to the small company with no in-house facilities for process development.

A totally integrated service for development chemistry is probably still not available, although a number of companies shown in Table 5.3 may provide something close. These companies do not necessarily provide production manufacture, although it is notable that some of these, such as Oxford Asymmetry (with Cambrex) and Albany

Table 5.2 Combinatorial chemistry providers and links to major pharmaceutical companies

Company	Major partner(s)	Relationship	Comments
3-D Pharmaceuticals	None as yet		Awarded broad patent in 1995 regarding combinatorial techniques
Affymax	Glaxo	Acquired	Peptide and non-peptide technology. One of the most established combinatorial chemistry companies
Alanex	Astra; Novo Nordisk; Roche	Research collaboration	Molecular design
ArQule	Pharmacia; Abbott; Roche; Solvay; T Cell Sciences	Strategic alliance	Solid phase and solution combinatorial chemistry expertise
Arris Pharmaceutical	Bayer; Pharmacia & Upjohn	Strategic alliance	Protease inhibitor specialisation. Lead tryptase inhibitor APC 366 in development for asthma
Chiron	Ciba; Organon	Partial tender (Ciba); research collaboration (Organon)	Technology transfer arrangement. Peptide diversity technology pooled with Houghten (below)
CombiChem	Teijin; Roche	Research collaboration	Versatile combinatorial technology provider. Variety of products and packages
Diversomer Technologies		None as yet	Proprietary technology and data handling techniques; derived from Parke Davis Research labs in Ann Arbor, MI

Company	Partners	Type	Description
Houghten Pharmaceuticals	e.g. Ribogene; Cadus; Osiris Therapeutics; Chromaxome; Novo Nordisk; Proctor and Gamble	Via contract	Proprietary technology. Agreement with Ribogene concerns anti-infectives and anti-cancer drugs with Cadus, acute inflammation; with Osiris Therapeutics, stem cell maturation
Isis Pharmaceuticals	Boehringer Ingelheim and others	Via contract	Research with Boehringer in field of adhesion molecules. In another project, a lead compound Isis 5320 has been identified for HIV therapy
Irori Quantum Microchemistry	Unknown	Via contract	Proprietary technology using encoded memory chips acting as electronic tag for the compound
Ixsys	Unknown	Via contract	Peptide and non-peptide technologies. Concerned with phage proteins. Therapeutic areas include cancer and ophthalmic conditions
Oncogene	BioChem Pharma	Research collaboration	
Oxford Diversity	Pfizer; LeukoSite	Strategic alliance	Broad-based generic technologies for combinatorial synthesis
Peptide Therapeutics	Alizyme	Via contract	Combinatorial chemistry; provision of libraries. Provision of RAPID™ lead discovery technology
Pharmacopeia	Schering Plough; Berlex; Sandoz; Organon	Strategic alliances/ research collaborations	Small molecule combinatorial synthesis for cancer, asthma (Schering-Plough) and multiple sclerosis (Berlex)

continued overleaf

Table 5.2 (continued)

Company	Major partner(s)	Relationship	Comments
PharmaGenics	Boehringer Mannheim	Strategic alliance	Research with Boehringer Mannheim towards restoration of tumour suppressive factor p53. PharmaGenics has own research interests in angiogenesis, cancer, HIV
David Sarnoff Research Centre	SmithKline Beecham	Strategic alliance	Microengineering and computer control of fluids expertise. Aim to build synthetic molecules on a business-card-sized chip
Selectide	Hoechst Marion Roussel	Acquisition	Solid phase synthesis and identification (deconvolution) techniques. Lead compound SEL 2096, an inhibitor of Factor Xa is in preclinical development for anti-coagulant and anti-thrombotic therapy
Signal Pharmaceuticals	Tanabe	Via contract	In addition to combinatorial chemistry technology, Signal also offers cellular and enzymatic assays for high-throughput screening using robotics
Sphinx	Lilly	Acquisition	Broad-based generic technologies for combinatorial synthesis
Versicor	None as yet		Subsidiary of Sepracor

Molecular Research (with SIPSY Chemical of France), have formed strategic alliances with chemical manufacturers in order to do so. Oxford Asymmetry claim to provide 'the complete chemical solution' based also on their expertise with combinatorial chemistry through their subsidiary Oxford Diversity.[77] Albany Molecular Research also have an interest in chemical discovery and have contracts with Astra and Hoechst Marion Roussel. Others such as Pharm-Eco have joined with Battelle, to provide a full range of chemistry, preclinical safety and toxicology, and registration support for drug leads. Chiroscience occupy an interesting position, having founded their business on the benefits of asymmetric synthesis of chiral compounds, and a surge in regulatory concern about optical enantiomerism. There is a deepening awareness of the developmental problems created by greater chirality in drug design,[79] and like Oxford Asymmetry, Chiroscience's name belies an increasing pragmatism as to the chemistry they perform. Despite their expertise in chiral synthesis, they can provide process development and pilot-plant scale work to the client's specifications, having recently bought an FDA-approved plant with this capability. They also have an interest in bringing products to the market, either single enantiomer versions of existing drugs, or innovative new chemical entities.

In another interesting development, Zeneca has highlighted the capabilities of its business unit, LifeSciences Molecules. The aim is for LifeSciences Molecules to work with more partners from the biotechnology industry, to supply both active ingredients and complex intermediates. In addition to the capacity for new technology such as chiral synthesis, the organisation has multikilogram or tonne capacity in GMP facilities. LifeSciences Molecules also has experience of making oligonucleotides, peptides and antibodies, which may represent a significant proportion of the drugs of the future; scale-up of this chemistry has presented a particular challenge to development chemists. One of LifeScience's component parts, Cambridge Research Biochemicals, has formed a partnership with Isis Pharmaceuticals to concentrate on gene-based drugs. This is an interesting example of a large company breaking off a business unit, and letting it free to collaborate with external organisations for business purposes. No longer is its only purpose to serve Zeneca in the production of fine chemicals. Rather, it is to maximise the utilisation of the resources, fixed investment and skills in a far broader sense. Where it sees a need to enlarge its expertise in a particular area, LifeSciences has chosen to use a collaboration with Isis pharmaceuticals rather than resort to developing in-house skills or looking elsewhere within Zeneca.

Table 5.3 Integrated chemical process development and scale-up companies

Company	Location	Country
Albany Molecular Research/SIPSY Chemicals	Albany, NY/Avrillé	US/Fr.
Chiroscience	Cambridge	UK
OREAD	Lawrence, KS	US
Oxford Asymmetry/Cambrex	Oxford/Rutherford, NJ	UK/US
Pharm-Eco	Lexington, MA	US
Ricerca	Painesville, OH	US

Clearly, the strength of small companies such as these lies in their adaptability, and awareness of laboratory-scale research, but their limitations in equipment and plant make large-scale work problematic. From the manufacturer's perspective, a link with a company that specialises in process development can bring in customers and maintain maximum use of their equipment. The link also allows a relationship of trust to develop, and facilitates technology transfer. As such, both sides benefit.

Beyond process development, there are a large number of chemical scale-up companies in the UK, US and elsewhere in Europe. The list shown in Table 5.4 is not intended to be complete, nor are the details of these companies provided. In some cases, the companies have potential to handle larger quantities; Chirex, for example, has the capacity to produce manufacturing scale quantities. Torcan has an affiliated relationship with a manufacturer, Delmar, that is in the vicinity. Each company in the table may have specific areas of expertise in terms of chemistry with which it is familiar, or hazardous work for which it has specialised handling equipment. Some are reticent about handling certain kinds of chemical hazard which in some cases is due to an incident that occurred in the past that they are anxious not to repeat. In other cases, there are environmental restrictions imposed by their local environmental regulations which prohibit certain chemicals.

Chemical manufacture is not a direct consideration during the preclinical stage of drug development. However, by the end of Phase II, it should be an objective to have in place a process that can be transferred into manufacture.[80] Ideally, there should be few if any changes to the process after entry into Phase III, though it may be inevitable that some small degree of fine-tuning is necessary on the way towards the pre-registration stage (and even beyond). The list of companies referred to in Table 5.5 is for guidance only: it is by no means comprehensive.

Table 5.4   *Scale-up providers (up to 10–50 kg)*

Company	Location	Country
BioDoc	Haverhill	UK
Cambridge Chemicals	Germantown, WI	US
Carbogen	nr Zurich	Switz
Chemserve	Manchester	UK
Chemsyn	Lenexa, KA	US
Chirex	Dudley	UK
Gateway	St Louis, MO	US
High Force	Durham	UK
International Science Center	Basle	Switz
Lancaster	Lancaster	UK
Melford	nr Ipswich	UK
Mitchell Cotts	W. Yorkshire	UK
Palmer Research Labs	Holywell	UK
QuChem	Belfast	UK
TCI	Portland, OR	US
Torcan	Aurora, Ontario	Can

Table 5.5   *Scale-up to chemical manufacture*

Company	Location	Country
Austin Chemical company	Buffalo Grove, IL	US
Bachem	Bubendorf	Switz
Celgene	Warren, NJ	US
Chemoxy	Middlesbrough	UK
Davos	Englewood Cliffs, NJ	US
Delmar	Montreal	Can
Eastman Fine Chemicals	Newcastle	UK
EMS-Dottikon	Dottikon	Switz
Finorga	Chasse sur Rhone	Fr
Hickson and Welch	Castleford	UK
IBIS Halebank	Widnes	UK
Laporte	Middlesbrough	UK
Lonza	Basle	Switz
Macfarlan Smith	Edinburgh	UK
Newport	Dublin	Ireland
Orgamol	Evionnaz	Switz
PPG Industries	Pittsburgh, PA	US
Robinson Brothers	West Bromwich	UK

5.2.2   Automated methods and high-throughput screening

As described in section 1.2.2, automation and high-throughput screening represent logical sequelae to combinatorial chemistry, and the technology in this area is advancing rapidly. It is true that much of the primary biochemical testing of combinatorial libraries is performed in large pharmaceutical companies, wherein the data will be used for in-house drug discovery projects. However, developments are taking place extremely rapidly, with the traditional 96-well plate being replaced by more dense formats for testing. At the end of 1996, the trend to use of the 384-well plate is underway, but on the horizon further advances to designs of up to 3000 wells per plate are being considered. Reducing the assay volume reduces costs of components, and such reductions are aimed towards miniaturisation to the region of one microlitre per assay. High-throughput assays have potential beyond initial biochemical screening, for other steps in the drug discovery and development process, such as stability, toxicity, bioavailability, metabolism, pharmacokinetics and pharmacodynamics. Because of these facts, and because it represents virgin territory for some companies, collaborations with external bodies have been a route that many have chosen to follow.

There is probably much potential for small companies as specialist providers of high-throughput screening technology. Aurora Biosciences' expertise in fluorescence screening has rapidly become popular for research collaborations (e.g. BMS, ArQule, Sequana, Alanex). It is possible that the extent of small company involvement in high-throughput screening will increase similarly to the situation in combinatorial chemistry, although at present it is much more typical for the screening of externally provided compounds to be conducted in-house.

The association of screening techniques with combinatorial chemistry has developed to a stage that allows the automated feedback of the results from the former into an iterative procedure with the latter. Two companies that are working on this technology are Neurogen and 3-Dimensional Pharmaceuticals (3DPC). In 1995, the latter received grant of a broad patent which covers the automatic generation of drug leads through computer-controlled robotic synthesis and structure activity analysis of test results. This perhaps represents the apotheosis of the computer in drug discovery. The irony is that it is based on semi-rational, iterative processes of drug discovery similar to the traditional methods that have delivered success over the years. It is not based on *a priori* prediction from principles of biological structure as was the hope for computer-generated drug design in the early 1970s.

The data produced by combinatorial synthesis and high-throughput screening techniques can be staggering compared to that traditionally produced in drug discovery projects. Daily screening rates of 50 000 (Glaxo Wellcome) or 100 000 compounds (Aurora) are possible in 1996. Traditional data entry techniques have had to be substantially modified to cope with this increase in workload. A number of partnerships have been formed for the specific purpose of handling the data generated. Glaxo Wellcome's relationship with Oxford Molecular has been dealt with elsewhere (see section 2.8). The aim of this collaboration is to allow the automatic generation of quantitative structure activity relationships from raw data without the intervention of the bench scientist. Tripos is a company well versed in this area, that is working with Merck on information services related to combinatorial chemistry and high-throughput screening; they have recently launched a consultancy service to address the structural diversity, data handling and analysis issues related to combinatorial chemistry. Molecular Design Limited and Chemical Design[81] are other companies that offer software packages or consultancy support in this area.

On the automation side, there is an increasing number of specialist companies offering a range of services in high-throughput screening. Examples of the services offered include:

- execution of high-throughput screening (in the range of 10 000 to 100 000 compounds)
- implementation of bioassays and optimisation for screening
- consulting services for setting up in-house services, robotics and automation, and acquisition of libraries

Examples of companies active in this field include Bureco, Robbins Scientific and Brandel. In the UK, a partnership between the Cruciform project (see p. 114) and The Automation Partnership has been awarded grant funding from the Department of Trade and Industry's Foresight Challenge programme. This is an interesting combination of biochemical expertise (Cruciform) and engineering capability (Automation Partnership) which will work with compounds supplied by combinatorial techniques from the US company Tripos. In the US, Axiom Biotechnologies has set up to provide high-throughput *in vitro* pharmacological screening based on automated measurement of physiological responses of target cells to test compounds. The system works using natural cells rather than the molecular biological constructs that employ reporter genes, as discussed in section 1.2.3.

From these considerations, it should be clear that the conduct of a modern, high-throughput assay for drug discovery based either on libraries generated by combinatorial chemistry or from natural sources should be feasible employing almost entirely out-of-house resources.

5.2.3   Biology

5.2.3.1   Molecular biology and biochemistry

Although combinatorial chemistry is perhaps the most favoured theme for alliances and collaborations amongst the major pharmaceutical industry companies, there is a substantial interest in other areas. Notable among these are those of gene therapy and genome analysis. Much of the science that underpins this technology was until recently classified as fundamental research carried out in academia, and the importance of basic work has been preserved in many of the commercial ventures, albeit in a focused way. The rapid progress in this science has largely been made outside the mainstream pharmaceutical industry, and most of the platform technology has been developed in the biotechnology sector. Once it became apparent that the cutting-edge science from these extramural laboratories could be assimilated into commercially important research for large pharma, it was inevitable that partnerships would be formed. The structure for the deals has been similar to that described in section 5.2.1.2, with payments made upfront and on the basis of actual work done (full-time equivalents of scientists), together with milestone payments and royalties for any products that reach the market. In addition, issues relating to intellectual property need to be considered, and in this respect the reader is referred to the imaginative arrangement that was established between Alizyme and Peptide Therapeutics, described in section 6.6.

As mentioned earlier in more detail (see section 2.3), the human genome project will bring enormous amounts of data for consideration as the bases for novel therapeutic approaches. In addition to straight sequencing data, increasing attention is being directed to the function of gene products. One company with this in mind is Genetics Institute, which has a proprietary genomics programme called DiscoverEase to focus on functional genomics which is designed to be accessible by multiple partners. Most of the small companies in genomics have formed partnerships with one or more major pharmaceutical collaborators. In addition to these research technology-based arrangements, some attention is also being devoted to the substantial technical problems that arise in the purification and scale-up to production of gene therapy vectors. One company offering consultancy on this and other issues related to the pharmaceutical aspects of gene therapy is AEA Technology, based in Didcot in the UK. Some of the companies in this area are shown in Table 5.6. This is not meant to be an exhaustive analysis of the partnerships in this field, since such data are practically out of date before they are written. The table serves to indicate the range of partnerships available, and that it has become the norm rather than the exception for small research companies of this kind to engage in alliances or collaborative arrangements with major pharmaceutical partners. There is every indication that this trend will continue.

As with combinatorial chemistry, there is a heavy emphasis for companies providing research in this area to be based in the US. One of the factors behind this trend is the more favourable environment for patenting of DNA sequences in the US (and Japan) relative to Europe. European Union policy on the issue of intellectual property for genetically modified organisms, as represented by the saga of the oncomouse (see section 5.2.3.2), has been to vacillate in the face of ecological, environmental and ethical pressure to resist technological change. This has produced an aura of uncertainty that has done the business environment no good.

One further reason for the pre-eminence of the US in this area has been the availability of substantial amounts of public money from the National Institutes of Health (NIH). However, the funds for basic science in the US from government sources are now declining, and expected to decline further as a result of budget-balancing initiatives which accord basic science less priority than Medicare and social security. There are moves in the US to restrict the Small Business Innovation Research (SBIR) grants available from the NIH to the biotechnology industry, although the level of grants seems to have been preserved, at least for fiscal 1997. In fiscal 1995, this system has supplied over $200m to emerging biotechnology companies, and a statutory set-aside is imposed on federal research budgets for SBIR grants. Whatever the outcome for these moves in the US, it is clear that world-wide restrictions on government-funded research are being forced by legislators' desires to limit public spending in general; science is seen as the soft political option.

Although most of these collaborations are between companies of greatly different sizes, alliances between small companies are becoming increasingly common. Examples from Table 5.6 include that between Sequana and Aurora Biosciences. Using the combination of expertise, the two companies are able to consider joint discovery programmes. In the example quoted, Sequana will analyse the function of disease genes while Aurora will provide ultra-high-throughput screening technology employing fluorescent techniques. Arrangements

Table 5.6 *Partnerships in molecular biology*

Minor partner	Major partner	Technology	Relationship
Allelix	Lilly	Neurochannel cloning	Research collaboration
Applied Immune Sciences	Rhône Poulenc Rorer	Gene therapy	Acquired
Cantab	Pfizer	DISC-virus viral design	Research collaboration
Clontech	Roche	Gene target identification	Research collaboration
GeneMedicine	Corange	Gene therapy	Research collaboration
Genetic therapy	Sandoz	Gene therapy	Acquired
Genovo	Biogen	Gene therapy	Research collaboration
Gilead	Glaxo Wellcome	Gene therapy	Research collaboration
Gryphon	Therexsys	Gene therapy	Research collaboration
Hexagen	None as yet	Functional genomics	
ICOS	Glaxo Wellcome	Genomic analysis and gene expression (PDE enzymes)	Research collaboration
Immusol	Pfizer	Gene therapy	Research collaboration
Incyte	Hoechst Marion Roussel/ Upjohn/Zeneca/Pfizer	Genome analysis/ bioinformatics	Research collaboration
Isis	Novartis	Antisense anti-cancer	Research collaboration/co-development; Isis have also formed a collaboration with ProtoGene laboratories for automation equipment

Joslin Medical Centre	Boehringer Mannheim	Gene therapy	Research collaboration
Lynx Therapeutics	Hoechst Marion Roussel/Upjohn	Genome analysis	Research collaboration
Microcide	Pfizer	Gene target identification	Research collaboration
Millennium	Astra/Roche/Lilly/American Home Products	Gene therapy	Research collaboration
Myriad Genetics	Novartis	Genome analysis	Research collaboration
Neurocrine	Novartis	Altered peptide ligands	Research collaboration
Oxford University/Wellcome Trust	Zeneca/Merck	Genome analysis	Research collaboration
Progenitor	Chiron	Gene therapy	Acquired
RPMS Technology	SmithKline Beecham	Signature-tagged mutagenesis	Research collaboration
Sequana	Boehringer Ingelheim/Corange/Glaxo Wellcome/Aurora Biosciences	Genome analysis	Research collaboration
Sibia	Lilly	Receptor clones	Research collaboration
Somatix therapy	Squibb	Gene therapy	Research collaboration
Synaptic	Lilly	Receptor cloning	Research collaboration

like this are likely to become more common as the range of specialities exemplified within the biotechnology sector becomes broader.

The popularity of genomic science for research collaborations is huge currently encompassing 40% of large pharma. Some of the more advanced companies in this field have been able to derive substantial incomes from collaborations. For example, Millennium in 1995 recorded fees of nearly $23m which enabled the company to post a net income, as opposed to a net loss, which is the normal financial result for companies operating in this or similar fields. It should be noted that the fees recorded in Millennium's accounts are for monies actually received. Much of the glamour surrounding research collaborations based on figures of tens of millions of dollars assumes that milestone payments and royalties will become due at some time in the future. In fact the actual payments made at the start of a collaboration are normally substantially less. The fact that Millennium made a profit based on payments for work done rather than results achieved is perhaps indicative of the attractiveness of the technology provider as opposed to the research product provider (see section 5.3). Thus the acquisition of the technology was a major factor behind Chiroscience's takeover of Darwin Molecular.

Collaborations in this field are rapidly changing. For a reasonably up-to-date picture, the reader is referred to the growing information available on the World Wide Web.[28]

5.2.3.2   *Pharmacology*

Pharmacology is a core discipline that has historically been conducted almost exclusively in-house, and in close association with other disciplines. It is also a core discipline in the sense that it is crucial to pharmaceutical R&D, and will remain so despite the changes that have occurred in discovery processes.

Unlike the earlier subjects such as combinatorial chemistry and genomics, technological expertise in pharmacology is widespread and growing much less rapidly. Moreover, pharmacological techniques and results are discussed much more openly than many other aspects of the discovery of a drug. This is because these techniques and results are largely considered unpatentable. The common form of alliances discussed in sections 5.2.1.2 and 5.2.3.1 involves some arrangement concerning intellectual property. This form of alliance is therefore rarely open for partnerships involving pharmacology.

Despite the above comments, patent applications are increasingly being made for biochemical modes of action as the basis for therapy of certain disease states. As an example, Merck recently applied for a patent (GB 2 288 733A) for adenosine A3 antagonists useful as anti-allergics or anti-inflammatories based on their activity as suppressors of eosinophil function. Whether this particular patent issues survives the examination process intact remains to be seen, but the existence of other examples suggests that the principle of the use of patents to cover pharmacological advances is gaining ground.

The value of these new types of patent application to a technological provider of pharmacology services is based both on grant of the application, and on finding a successful means of marketing that intellectual property. Inventors of pharmacological techniques or models may not be able to claim ownership of land bounded by the same rigid fences as inventors of composition of matter; their claims may be seen more as signposts of expertise that others may use at a cost.

The incursion of molecular biological techniques into pharmacology has spawned the production of transgenic animals that have been the subject of some celebrated patent applications around the world. Most famous is Harvard University's oncomouse, for which a patent application was made, claiming the incorporation of a human oncogene into a mammalian genome to produce cancer in a mammal. This patent was issued in the US, but is still being considered by the European Patent Office, and is the subject of intense debate in the patenting community. As a result of the continuing uncertainty about the patent protection surrounding the oncomouse, together with the exclusion of use for research purposes from Harvard's rights, many other pharmaceutical companies have developed their own expertise in transgenic models of cancer. These represent proprietary models for investigation of a disease. Even if a patent does ensue, the strategy of applying for one may not have yielded the best outcome for Harvard University. An alternative approach may have been to offer the breed of mouse in a controlled way to preferred clients, under a framework that maintained Harvard's technological lead and at the same time brought in funds to enable future research. A similar business proposition applies for other organisations with transgenic animals, given the long-term nature of development of such models, which if widely used may become standard tests for novel therapeutics in certain areas.

Perhaps in line with this sentiment, partnerships with pharmacology providers based on contractual arrangements are increasing, although from a small base. Pharmacology is a specialised discipline in which valuable expertise is built up over many years. This expertise is associated, for instance, with certain areas within pharmacology and particularly with specialised animal models. An example could be CNS pharmacology, in which the measurement of outcome, use of a precise protocol and establishment of a steady baseline response and/

or standard drug effect can take many months of practice and years of prior training in associated techniques. Examples of organisations which provide a contractual source for CNS pharmacology as well as other specialisations are shown in Table 5.7.

Table 5.7 also shows contract providers of general pharmacology such as Panlabs, who have recently signed an agreement with Tripos to provide a composite package of services including combinatorial chemistry and computerised techniques of molecular modelling and data handling. This represents one of the first entire drug discovery packages available on a contractual basis.

As we consider the further use of pharmacology in a developmental setting, safety pharmacology is routinely conducted in the environment of a CRO. In this case, the reasons for outsourcing are closely associated with those for outsourcing toxicology, such as accommodation of bulges in workload, and some of the providers of this service can be found in section 5.2.4.

5.2.3.3   *Pharmaceutics*

Consideration of the physicochemical properties of a drug candidate is not as glamorous as some of the more basic components of drug discovery, and has often been given too little attention. A wide number of CROs can conduct this work under the direction of a drug's discovery partner, although the majority of large pharmaceutical companies also routinely perform it in-house. Examples of organisations with specific expertise in pharmaceutics include Applied Analytical Industries (AAI) and OREAD in the US and Aston Molecules in the UK.

As a consequence of the stricter regulatory environment in pharmaceutics, some large pharmaceutical companies have constructed (Glaxo Wellcome, Zeneca) or are constructing (SmithKline Beecham, Pfizer) facilities to state-of-the-art specifications. They may turn out to be too large or too small for ongoing programmes (not dissimilar from the overcapacity in other areas such as toxicology pathology facilities mentioned earlier), for it is impossible to plan for what might be in development throughout the lifetime of the facility. There will be times when in-house resources will be inadequate and resources must be provided externally. Equally there will be times when the internal resources are underutilised. As the pressure builds on R&D budgets, and outsourcing becomes increasingly favoured, R&D management of large companies may question whether this highly regulated low-to-medium technology is part of their core activities.

Certainly, investment in such facilities is not an option for the small, emerging research-based biopharmaceutical companies. These

Table 5.7 Contract pharmacology providers

Name	Specialisation	Location	Country
Battelle	Respiratory/General	Geneva	Switzerland
Bio-Pharma-Simon	General	Wavre	Belgium
BioResearch Laboratories		Montreal	Canada
CERB	CNS/General	Baugy	France
Cerebrus	CNS	Ascot, Berks	UK
Coromed	Cardiovascular	Albany, NY	US
Field Pharma	Pharmacology Profiling	Vizcaya	Spain
HTI Bioservices	Large animal specialists; surgical/cardiovascular	San Diego, CA	US
Huntingdon Life Sciences	General	Huntingdon	UK
ITEM Labo	CNS	Cedex	France
Neurotech	General	Geneva	Switzerland
Neurotrack	Pharmacology Profiling	Royal Holloway & Bedford New College, Egham	UK
Northview Bioservices	Rodent pharmacology	Berkeley, CA	US
Nova	Biochemistry Profiling	Baltimore, MD	US
Oread BioSafety Center	Safety Pharmacology	Lawrence, KS	US
Panlabs	Pharmacology Profiling	Bothell, WA	US
Pharmagene	Human tissue specialists	Royston	UK
Quintiles	Respiratory/CV/CNS	Edinburgh	UK
RCC, Geneva	Respiratory	Geneva	Switzerland
Rephartox	Pharmacology Profiling	Marssen	Netherlands
TNO Pharma	Respiratory	Zeist	Netherlands
TSI Mason/Genzyme	General	Worcester, MA	US
Will Labs	General	Ashland, OH	US
William Harvey Research Institute	Cardiovascular/Inflammation	London	UK

companies need to be expertly serviced by contract organisations that can provide formulation, stability testing and manufacture of clinical grade materials. With regard to the latter capability it will be important to include the sterile formulation of parenteral biological materials.

The stricter regulatory environment of pharmaceutics makes it appropriate for outsourcing on a contractual basis, but it is not an area that can be managed in the traditional manner of toxicology. Formulation programmes can be very open-ended and difficult to plan. This must be understood at the outset, with the contract being set up to account for the effort put into the project rather than for achieving success. Considering the points made earlier about highly potent compounds having the physicochemical properties of grease balls or brick dust (see p. 31) it is also important for everyone, especially the client, to have realistic expectations. Pharmaceutical development expertise can rarely turn a sow's ear into a silk purse.

There are a number of more sophisticated ways in which the pharmacodynamic properties of the drug entity can be altered by techniques of formulation, and a number of companies who specialise in this area. Companies such as Alza (California) and Elan* (Ireland) have formed partnerships with larger companies to control the delivery of a drug candidate to fit the ideal clinical and marketing requirements. The advantages of such manipulation include longer dosing intervals, leading to greater patient compliance, and maintenance of steadier blood levels, leading to fewer side-effects. Alza in particular have been very successful in forming over 20 partnerships with a great many of the major international pharmaceutical companies. Historically, these companies have also typically applied drug delivery technology to drugs that are on the market already in order to improve their characteristics in terms of dosing frequency. Napp and its associated companies Mundipharma and Purdue Frederick have preferred not to engage in partnerships, but have successfully brought off-patent drugs through to the market in controlled release forms. The commercial gains from this (relatively straightforward) means to improve a drug's therapeutic attraction are often quite pronounced, and this has been commented on before (see section 1.2.3).

The greater acceptance and availability of measures to control release from formulation of medicines suggests that it may be used more widely, and earlier in drug development. Rather than discarding short-acting compounds, and referring the problem back to the iterative cycle of the medicinal chemist and biological evaluation,

---

* Now merged with Athena Neurosciences to combine the delivery and discovery strengths of the two companies.

controlled release versions of drugs may be suitably developed. A once-daily or twice-daily therapy is being increasingly expected by both the patient and the practitioner, which means that this technology can be valuably applied during development to intercept the appearance of normal release versions that would require more frequent administration. Alza, at least, is looking to form partnerships with this in mind. Elan has chosen an alternative strategy recently in deciding to merge with Athena, perhaps with the aim of employing their proprietary technology to control the properties of internal drug development candidates.

The recent interest in biological products for human therapeutic use, such as active compounds based on a peptidic or oligonucleotide structure, has increased the importance of new drug delivery technology. Indeed, the poor bioavailability characteristics of such molecules has given rise to the suggestion that lack of oral bioavailability represents the 'Achilles' heel of the biotechnology industry'.[82] Various new approaches to getting the active moiety to the site of action are being intensively investigated, such as the use of liposomes, or carriers based on lipophilic elements that are cleaved at the site of action. The liposome approach has been applied for example to the delivery of amphotericin B, for antifungal therapy. A number of companies have been involved in this work, including Sequus, NeXstar and the Liposome Company in the US. Using the pro-drug approach, Bodor and colleagues have successfully used a cholesteryl ester to deliver enkephalin to the CNS; once inside, ester cleavage reveals a modified enkephalin peptide which is impermeant to the blood–brain barrier, and is trapped in the CNS where it can exert a pharmacological effect.[83] Elegant solutions to circumvent the body's natural barriers are particularly needed for gene therapy, in which delivery of genetic material across gut, cellular and nuclear membranes is required. Although viral vectors have been investigated in the past, much attention is currently being directed towards 'softer' non-biological mechanisms of gene delivery, as evidenced by the work of companies such as GeneMedicine, Therexys and Megabios. In the absence of such solutions the eventual therapy is either going to be poorly effective, or at best, will require relatively unpleasant administration regimes. For instance, Alza are applying their osmotic mini-pump for delivery directly into the CNS of Ribozyme's products for CNS disease.

Entry into the body other than through the mouth is being considered for a variety of drugs, such as by transdermal passage. Although there are some advantages for selected molecules delivered by this route, the skin was designed by nature to be impermeable (it is also surprisingly powerful in metabolising xenobiotics), and this route is only really applicable to drugs which are very potent, quite lipophilic and relatively water-soluble. A good example is nicotine. The transdermal route is of course also useful for drugs designed for topical therapy. The use of the lung for systemic delivery also represents one option for potent peptides and proteins that would normally be broken down in the inimical environment of the stomach and upper intestinal tract, and this is a subject that Andaris is pursuing in the UK; this route also offers potential for delivery of gene products, such as for cystic fibrosis. Colonic delivery is another approach, since this route offers the opportunity to avoid the first-pass metabolism of the liver. A summary of some of the smaller companies active in this field, their relationships with larger partners and particular scientific approach is given in Table 5.8.

Drug delivery approaches can enable the fast-track development of therapies with lower exposure to risk than the conventional approach of small molecules for oral delivery. For instance, Guildford Pharmaceuticals is rare among the biotechnology community, in being a company with a product that has been recently approved by the FDA for treatment of brain tumours. The product, gliadel, is a slow-release biodegradable polymer wafer that contains the chemotherapy agent carmustine (BCNU). Release of the drug over a three-month period knocks out any remaining tumour cells after surgery, without the side-effects that ensue from systemic exposure to the toxic effects of carmustine. Clinical trials have suggested a decrease in 12-month mortality of 44%. Guildford could be in profit by 1998, a facet shared by only 8 of the 200 or so US biotechnology companies. It is also rare among biotechnology companies in choosing to go it alone to the market, at least in the US; the company may well seek partners for marketing in other continents. It is also worth mentioning Core Technologies, based in Scotland, that specifically offers controlled-release technology to companies with compounds that are currently in later development.

Despite the advantages in terms of easier commercialisation, for companies to remain successful in this area requires maintenance of a technological lead over the competition. The wheel of invention may turn faster to the benefit of commercial return, but it turns at the same rate for the competition too.

5.2.4   Toxicology and ADME studies

Toxicology is bread and butter business for CROs and the choice is sufficiently wide for its repetition in this work to be superfluous. Of all the disciplines for outsourcing, toxicology is the most popular

Table 5.8 Drug delivery collaborations

Company	Approach	Major partner(s)
Access Pharmaceuticals Inc	Bioresponsive smart polymer systems	None as yet
Alkermes	Microparticular controlled release	Boehringer Mannheim/Schering Corp
Alza	Transdermal and controlled release oral formulations	Various
Andaris	Systemic pulmonary delivery of proteins and peptides	None as yet
Cortecs	Oral peptide and protein delivery	Osteometer (Denmark)
DanBioSyst	Various delivery systems for biopharmaceuticals	Lilly/Janssen/Sandoz/Wyeth-Ayerst and others
Elan	Transdermal and controlled release oral formulations	Various
Elite laboratories	Oral controlled release formulations	Celgene
Flamel	Controlled release microencapsulation	Bristol Myers Squibb/Searle/SB
Focal	Biodegradable drug delivery for restenosis	Chiron
Inex Pharmaceuticals	Intracellular gene delivery	Schering Plough
LTS Technologies	Microemulsion technology	None as yet
	Transdermal technology	
Medtronic	Implantable pumps for diseases such as Huntingdon's	Regeneron
Megabios	Lipid/plasmid or DNA complexes for gene therapy	Pfizer/Glaxo Wellcome
ML Laboratories	Microcapsule drug delivery technology, e.g. for respiratory drugs	Glaxo Wellcome
PolyMASC	Pharmaceuticals coupled to polyethylene glycol	None as yet
Quadrant	Stabilisation of biopharmaceuticals (e.g. vaccines) using trehalose	Chiron Biocine
The Liposome Company	Liposome and other lipid-based drug delivery systems	Pfizer
Theratech	Transdermal patch technology	Proctor & Gamble/SB/Pfizer
Therexsys	Non-viral targeted gene delivery	None as yet
Vaxcel	Vaccine delivery	Corixa

among sponsors, with over 50% of all such studies conducted by contract extramurally. The reader is referred to the Technomark[52] or Soteros[53] directories for details of providers.

The nature of many of the toxicology studies lends them ideally to being done by contract. Although there may be no such thing as a routine study, there is a close resemblance between studies on different drugs; the regularity of the need for them from a sponsor's point of view is unpredictable, and maintaining in-house staff for peak demand is clearly inefficient. They can be reliably planned, for defined lengths of time, and there are distinct advantages in offering these kinds of services to a number of clients. Moreover, they are often long term, more predictable in their running and require less monitoring than, say, pharmacology studies. CROs have gathered substantial expertise in toxicology, and the value of this can sometimes be overlooked. CROs are keen to point out their specialist expertise and planning capabilities in terms of offering a service which includes more than one study. There may be particular advantages to a small company in making use of packaged services, especially as this may include advice on regulatory matters and aspects for later development.

There are some specialist providers which deserve a mention. The Celltox Centre is set in the academic environment of the University of Hertfordshire. It has been specifically interested in the establishment of *in vitro* methods of toxicological evaluation which have found favour in the light of the increasing concerns for animal welfare. Despite limited success in the discovery of an alternative for the notorious Draize eye test in rabbits (see p. 124), interest in cellular alternatives remains high on the public's agenda for change in the methods used in drug discovery.

In the earlier evaluation of potential drug candidates, the increasing use of *in vitro* metabolism in liver is a service offered by most major CROs. Conducting these studies at ever earlier stages is suggested as a means of predicting the outcome of more expensive whole animal studies; in addition, these studies can be performed on greater numbers of candidates. A more recent technique involves passage through cultured CACO 2 cells as a measure of absorption. The increasing demand for it is suggested by the recent appearance on the scene of In Vitro Technologies (Baltimore, MD).

5.2.5   Clinical studies and registration

For late development, some of the activities that are required will include clinical studies and registration, which have not been given a great deal of attention in this book, the aim being to concentrate on preclinical development. Clinical studies are routinely conducted in a hospital setting, and the co-ordination of these studies through to the acquisition and statistical interpretation of data is a core activity of many CROs. The aptitude of the major CROs is being increasingly recognised by the major pharmaceutical companies, since their experience in terms of the number of clinical trials that they manage is rarely surpassed. Their global presence and experience in handling recruitment of large numbers of patients often make these organisations a preferred choice over internally co-ordinated studies if rapid regulatory submission is a prime factor. Quintiles, one of the major world-wide CROs, has grown rapidly in the last few years from a base of statistical evaluation. One may argue that this is *the* core technology of CROs that operate in clinical trials, with application in many other fields of CROs' activities. Examination of the involvement of CROs in the clinical area suggests that the bulk of the work concerns Phase II–IV studies (60%), with Phase I occupying 20% and data management and statistics 15%; regulatory and other work relates to 5% of activities.[52]

Registration is increasingly a popular topic for consultancies, and their use for this is growing. There are of course regulatory departments within large CROs that can give the client the benefit of their experience across a number of different drug development projects. There are also numerous small consultancies that offer specialist regulatory advice for the markets of interest to their clients.

5.3   SMALL, MULTIDISCIPLINARY RESEARCH COMPANIES OR TECHNOLOGY PROVIDERS?

Although there is a general shift of pharmaceutical R&D towards out-of-house work at many kinds of institution, the greatest growth is currently to be found in the small start-up companies. This diverse collection has been grouped by the misnomer 'biotechnology' to describe its activities. The scope of the definition seems to include niche technology providers of combinatorial chemistry or genomics, which have little to do with the historic provenance of the term as it related to companies such as Amgen or Genentech, who produced biological products. Biotechnology has also been applied to human diagnostic or agricultural use, in addition to therapeutic purposes, although this discussion will be restricted to the latter category.

In many cases, biotechnology companies provide whole research programmes. In 1995, the total number of research projects being carried out in such companies was equal to the number being carried out in medium and large companies.[84] The variety of therapeutic targets, and of approaches to these targets, together with the speed at which the field is changing makes a complete overview of this field impossible within the confines of this book. However, rather than giving a detailed analysis of every biotechnology company and its partner profile, there are some general principles which underpin the field. Philosophically, there is a substantial difference between outsourcing a component of a research project, or a development project, and outsourcing the entire discovery process. One major part of that difference is that the creative process is also outsourced, and with it the basic patent rights (see also section 6.6). The biotechnology partner will probably already have established a patent position with regard to the biochemical nature of the target, an assay system to screen for activity (particularly if the system has been genetically engineered) and maybe even a (number of) lead compound(s). Issues of prior intellectual property rights may be a feature of some of the more mature partnerships involving combinatorial chemistry or genomics, where these companies have filed patent applications, but this is the exception rather than the rule. In the case of technologically-based partnerships, these patents are not usually related to a drug entity in the therapeutic area of interest. In partnerships focusing on a target-based R&D project, intellectual property rights such as to the drug entity itself, such patents are normally retained by the original (biotechnology company) inventor who may licence them to a partner.

The issue of a strong patent position is one of the major assets of a small company, and as was the case with Cetus, can in itself contribute significantly to its commercial value. Cetus was assigned the rights to the polymerase chain reaction (PCR), a critical technique in modern molecular biology, for which its inventor Kary Mullis received the Nobel Prize in 1993. After Chiron bought Cetus, it sold the entire patent portfolio to Roche for $300m. The ability of a small company to raise money can be significantly influenced by patent applications, and although the PCR example points to the ability to patent techniques rather than products, this is an exception rather than the rule. Broad patents filed by technology providers in areas such as genomics and combinatorial chemistry will need to withstand litigative onslaught (as did the PCR patent), and will require constant surveillance to pre-empt and attack unauthorised use of the invention. Research project providers aim to obtain rights to products which can prove the basis for future therapies. As mentioned earlier (see section 2.3.1), venture capital and stock market analysts are likely to regard investment in therapy-targeted companies more sympathe-tically, partly because of the greater security and value of their intellectual property.

The component parts of a deal involving a target-based R&D project are similar to those described in section 5.2.1.2, that is upfront and equity payments, R&D costs, milestone and royalty payments. The rate for these components for a number of deals has been reviewed,[28] and the average rate for royalties is similar to those for the technology-provider partnerships (6–10%), but the overall level of the other payments is about a third less, totalling $25.4m. One may conclude from this that the present frenetic rate of negotiating in the areas of combinatorial chemistry and genomics has created a situation in which a premium is being paid for these services. This premium is not available in general for collaborative deals based on complete projects. The potential for this to change if one type of approach becomes assessed as most likely to succeed in clinical and commercial terms, must be tempered by the fact that these deals are usually struck at a research stage, and if sufficient clinical work has been done on a competitor compound to prove the concept, the rewards for a successor three to four years behind are unlikely to be very tempting.

For a small company to offer research collaborations effectively to a larger partner, attractiveness of the package on offer must be based largely on a highly creative and competent scientific research effort. The situation is somewhat different if a small company offers the results of its endeavours for licence at the end of Phase I or Phase II evaluation. In that case, the large company is paying for what has been achieved rather than what it expects to be accomplished.

The fact that a large company may consider outsourcing the entire discovery process suggests that it is not burdened with undue hubris as to its ability to conduct such work in-house. The environment for such outsourcing is a good deal more fertile than it was a few years ago. Large companies are recognising that they may have some elements to learn from small company methods, perhaps along the lines of those factors mentioned in chapter 2. However, there are substantial disadvantages too, and in drug discovery as a totality, the integrative characteristics and historical experience of large companies are some of their major strengths. For all the criticism of the large pharmaceutical companies as 'lumbering giants', giants they remain, and they have not been slow to recognise the importance of new technology in drug discovery. Despite the existence of small com-panies as high-class providers of such technology, the biggest companies such as Glaxo Wellcome and Merck have produced combinatorial chemistry and high-throughput screening programmes that are second to none. The economies of scale when operating a large number of screens for therapeutic targets have made the application of the latest, best, and often the most expensive technology cost-effective, in a way not possible at smaller outfits.

For these reasons, small companies offering research project collaborations need to couple them with a specific novel therapeutic target, expertise, or history of success which makes the reasons for entering into these arrangements self-evident. A large company needs to be persuaded of the wisdom of outsourcing a particular research project because the small company offers, say, a more flexible and conducive environment to research, or access to specific target-related screens that would take too long to set up in-house. The small company needs to ensure that the integration of the biological and chemical research efforts is very close, and that their scientists are motivated to work hard as a team in order to share in the benefits of success. These facets which a small company may profess to offer as an advantage over their potential partner need to be offset by the breadth of experience and greater access to any and all facilities that pertain in the larger companies.

In the next decade or two it may become normal for research to be conducted in small companies (as described in chapter 6) and development in large ones. If this becomes accepted practice, it will coincide with the maturation of such small companies (who may no longer be small at all), generation of track records and the recognition of some of them as centres of excellence. Alongside this development, some companies will inevitably fail. The question is, which?

One of the main reasons why companies are now emerging specifically with the objective of offering early stage research collaborations is that a previous generation of similar companies have successfully entered into co-development deals with their proprietary drugs at the end of Phase I or Phase II. Of course, going further back, the term 'biotechnology company' grew up with the likes of Amgen and Genentech, who were able to bring their own products right through to market and grow enormously as a result. Success of this kind challenged the belief within the large multinationals of their innate superiority in pharmaceutical R&D.

There is, theoretically, great value associated with the combination of multiple disciplines under one roof. The niche or specialist element to such an enterprise derives from the focus of research or therapeutic area. The multidisciplinary approach then offers a synergistic combination of activities. The argument for these synergies to be better provided on a small rather than large scale suggests that large pharmaceutical companies have not made full use of the possibilities for cross-fertilisation among multiple disciplines within them. Partly, this is a reflection of size, but it is also an indictment of their tendency to be organised on a departmental basis. Defenders of the departmental structure can point to the strength in single disciplines attained by this means. They can also point to the success of certain niche technology providers (as distinct from research project or research product providers), within the biotechnology sector.

The arguments for and against project-based and discipline-based structures have been long discussed within the pharmaceutical industry. Ultimately, there is value in both approaches, depending on the situation. For instance, in rapidly developing scientific areas there may be stronger arguments for single technology strengths than in more mature areas. Mature sciences have more to gain from fertilisation by associated disciplines, and from a multidisciplinary structure. In either case, and certainly where a mixture of these approaches is warranted, a small organisation has much to recommend it.

The philosophical difference between small multidisciplinary research companies and small single discipline technology providers extends to the type of partner they seek. Neither can aspire to supporting a complete pharmaceutical R&D effort, but each supplies a very different ethos. Small multidisciplinary research companies seek development capability and risk-buffers. It is rare to find this combination among CROs, although there are almost certain to be minor components of their work that small companies prefer to (or have to) contract out (see section 2.8). In addition, they seek co-development deals with large partners based on milestone payments and royalties. Their products are unlikely to reach commercial fruition for many years and their exposure to risk is high.

Single technology providers are experts within their field and may provide services purely on a contractual basis. Although these companies may be venture-capital based, their route to profitability is less tortuous; although small, they have many similarities to the larger CROs. Success depends upon selling technological excellence rather than selling a commercial drug candidate that has completed a Phase I or Phase IIa trial. Oxford Asymmetry is a single technology provider of chemical services. It has been in existence since 1992, and in 1995 returned its first profitable year. Longer established multidisciplinary providers have a more distant horizon for financial returns, since their profits are more dependent on registration and marketing of a new medicine. Many of the more mature companies in this arena have raised over $200m through venture capital and stock offerings; these amounts are in line with analyses of the amounts needed to progress a new molecular entity through to market (see section 2.1). These huge sums have been possible because of expectations that the eventual profits from such companies are likely to be much greater than those of a single discipline provider.

Some of the companies that were set up as single technology providers have been lured by the glamorous rewards of a blockbuster drug towards a more multidisciplinary basis. This strategy has both benefits and risks. The risks of drug discovery have been explicitly stated earlier, and the benefits are well known. The risks of the technological expert lie in a future that is difficult to predict, where the value of that technology is uncertain. The true importance of genomics or combinatorial chemistry to drug discovery is still unknown. But even if it is valuable, once it matures and becomes available to all, the advantage of a technological expert becomes increasingly difficult to discern. Under these circumstances, some might argue that the current penchant for outsourcing in these techniques may wane, and more work will be brought back into the large pharmaceutical companies.

There are suggestions that combinatorial chemistry will become a core technology in most pharmaceutical companies in a relatively short time—estimates vary from two to ten years. This indicates its rapid acceptance as a new technology for drug discovery; that although its worth is still to be established, the question is when, rather than if, it is useful. Technology providers need to consider how to maintain a lead, in order to differentiate themselves from other, similar companies. Product-based rather than technology-based providers are less prone to this long-term danger, in so far as they are differentiated on the value of the research into the therapeutic approach or on the drug candidate they can offer.

6
Towards the Virtual Research Company

In the present climate of change within the pharmaceutical industry, the question of strategy is a recurring theme. One approach is to create ever larger companies with greater global marketing muscle, the result of which upon the pharmaceutical industry in the past few years has been akin to radical surgery. Some of the surgery has been deconstructive, some constructive. Some of these changes will not have more than a cosmetic influence on the balance sheets of the companies concerned. However, surgery remains an apposite term in other ways, since the effects of these mergers, structural changes, dispositions and acquisitions are practically irreversible, for good or bad. On the other hand, the attraction of partnerships or other forms of co-operation is that if unsuccessful, they can be abrogated or otherwise modified to suit one or both partners.

Many of the collaborations in research with which this book deals are between large pharmaceutical companies and a smaller partner from industry or academia. For the large pharmaceutical company, such extramural collaborations, although growing, still only represent a minor portion of the way in which research is done. For instance, in 1994, Glaxo had 19 research alliances with small partners, and out-sourced £38m of research. Out of a total R&D spend in 1994 of around £800m, the proportion spent on extramural studies was relatively insignificant. (This contrasts with other claims from Glaxo in 1994 that 50% of toxicology and 25% of the R&D budget overall was spent extramurally; this figure is presumably influenced by a great deal of outsourced development work at CROs, which seemingly is more commonplace than outsourced research, although the latter is clearly also growing rapidly, primarily with partners from the biotechnology sector.) Zeneca reported 12 partnerships with biotechnology companies in 1995, which it planned to double in 1996. These figures for Glaxo in particular and the industry in general will have changed substantially in the last two years, and are likely to change further in the years to come, but the majority of activity in preclinical research will remain in-house for many years to come.

6.1   ALLIANCE CONSORTIA

Perhaps one of the most salient changes that is now taking place is represented by companies such as Pfizer and Rhône Poulenc Rorer (RPR) who have formed consortia of small biotechnology companies as a strategy for their research effort. RPR's group, called Gencell, currently includes 14 companies from the US and France, and is expected to enlarge to include Japanese companies too. The group is interested in cancer therapy, cardiovascular disease and central nervous system disorders, and is heavily biased towards gene therapy approaches using novel drug delivery technology (Table 6.1). Although there are few French companies in biotechnology as a whole, the alliance consortium reflects the national origins of RPR, and includes a number of Gallic components.

In this effort, RPR is leading the alliance consortium and co-ordinating the activities of the group. Dr Thierry Soursac, General Manager of Gencell, describes the efforts of the component companies as akin to suppliers of parts for an automobile manufacturer. Clearly, RPR hopes and expects to acquire a significant industry lead through this strategy. They have committed 200 RPR employees and $100m per year, or nearly 20% of the R&D budget on the venture. Their hopes for genomics are similar to those of SmithKline Beecham, who have also formed a smaller group of companies including Human Genome Sciences, the Virus Research Centre, Lark Technologies and Stanford University to provide this technology. These companies are combined with the David Sarnoff Research Institute and Orchid Biocomputer to provide combinatorial chemistry and molecular modelling capabilities.

Pfizer's efforts to build a network of biotechnology providers are known as PfizerGen (Table 6.2). This has been said to represent a strategic decision to position Pfizer for the next decade of drug discovery. Substantial financial investments of around $200m per year have been allocated to maintain such alliances, although the company stresses that these activities are designed to complement and not replace in-house research. This growth in research spending is also a

Table 6.1   Rhône Poulenc Rorer's alliance consortium, Gencell

Company	Location	Research focus
Rhône Poulenc Rorer	Fr.	Leader of alliance consortium
Genopoietic	Fr.	Anti-cancer
Introgen therapeutics	TX, US	Anti-cancer
Applied Immune Sciences	CA, US	Cell isolation technology
Darwin Molecular	WA, US	DNA sequencing
Lawrence Berkeley Human Genome Center	CA, US	DNA sequencing
Genethon	Fr.	Gene mapping and sequencing
Institut Pasteur, Lille	Fr.	High density lipoprotein cholesterol
CNRS	Fr.	Lipid-based vectors
Université Louis Pasteur	Fr.	Lipid-based vectors
Institut Gustav-Roussy	Fr.	Vector technology
Transgene	Fr.	Viral vectors
Virogenics	NY, US	Viral vectors
Genetix pharmaceuticals	NY, US	Retroviral cell packaging
Pasteur Merieux Connaught	Fr.	Vaccine technology

Table 6.2   The PfizerGen consortium 1996

Company	Location	Research focus
Incyte	CA, US	Gene therapy
Neurogen	CA, US	Neuroscience
Oncogene Sciences[a]	NY, US	Cancer therapy
Immusol	CA, US	Gene therapy (AIDS)
ChemGenics (formerly Myco)	MA, US	Antifungal discovery
AEA Technology	UK	Antisense technology
Oxford Diversity	UK	Combinatorial chemistry
Cambridge Antibody Technology	UK	Antibody technology
Cantab	UK	Recombinant vaccine technology
Microcide	CA, US	Anti-bacterial discovery
Cubist	MA, US	Combinatorial chemistry and drug design
Megabios	CA, US	Gene delivery
Bend	OR, US	Drug delivery technology

[a]   Pfizer has also invested in a project with Oncogene Sciences and New York University to develop treatments for baldness, wrinkles and pigment disorders.

reflection of the optimism for Pfizer's prospects for the future, based on its promising R&D pipeline. Again, genomics features prominently, along with screening automation, drug delivery and new therapeutic approaches external to Pfizer's existing portfolio.

One of these small companies, ChemGenics, was formed from the merger of Myco Pharmaceutical's drug discovery operations with

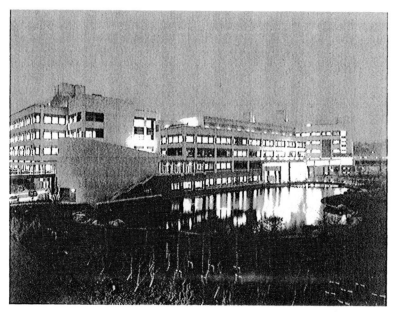

Figure 6.1   *Glaxo Wellcome's New Medicines Research Centre in Stevenage, UK*

PerSeptive Biosystems, another small company with expertise in drug development.

These examples represent a major change in research strategy beyond the simple one-to-one partnerships practised uniquely until very recently. Industrial and academic components find themselves increasingly rubbing shoulders. The role of the modern multinational pharmaceutical company is quite different from its traditional one, focusing increasingly on co-ordination and integration rather than operating with in-house technical expertise in parallel with the technology provider. How can we see this shift in functional terms, and what is the logical end-point for drug R&D?

6.2   ARCHITECTURE OF R&D

In the Introduction, the complex nature of drug R&D was compared to winning the Formula One Grand Prix Trophy. The complexity and difficulty of this project has dramatically increased in recent times. Both regulatory and medical pressures for safety and efficacy have increased the effort devoted to pharmaceutical R&D in large companies. A measure of these factors can be obtained by looking at the average number of pages in an NDA submission: this grew from 38 044 for the period 1977–80 to 90 650 for 1989–92; concomitant increases in the number of clinical trials and in patients per NDA were also observed in this period. Growth in the late 1980s in the industry produced huge emporia devoted to science, in which the multitudinous activities were usually placed in one site. Glaxo's monument to R&D, centralised at Stevenage in the UK (Figure 6.1), was completed in 1995 at a cost of practically $1bn, and at the time was the most expensive construction project in Europe, with the exception of the Channel Tunnel. One may conceptually draw these efforts as a single doric column, in which scientific departments align in close proximity. This is the diagrammatic representation of what has become known in business analytical circles as the FIPCO (fully integrated pharmaceutical company). The interplay between disciplines has been enhanced by propinquity, while the effort required to facilitate integration and co-ordination was minimised by this structure (Figure 6.2). Of course multidisciplinary co-operation can founder on interdepartmental rivalry and competition—even *schadenfreude*; but for the sake of this analogy, we will presume that it does work, as indeed it does in many large companies. The vertical dimension of the column is indicative of the timescale of the efforts that need to occur during the course of the discovery and development of a drug, with research at the bottom being succeeded by development above.

As the research and development effort becomes more difficult, the height and diameter of the column commensurately increases, representing the demonstrably greater resources required in the process. One has only to look at Glaxo's vast site to comprehend that huge infrastructure costs are associated with the in-house R&D effort. One is even more impressed from the inside, by the marble floors, the solid hardwood doors and the landscaped waterfalls. This is a substantial infrastructure from a substantial company, one with important economic implications for the UK in particular. The size of companies like Glaxo was important in the previous decades of industry growth, in persuading governments of the need for support in the form of realistic prices for their products. But today, such negotiations for new products can be very difficult, and the philosophical commitment of governments to pharmaceutical R&D at any price cannot be taken for granted. Changing the shape of the column is difficult without major efforts; its internal infrastructure is heavy and inflexible, and poorly suited to a rapidly changing scientific environment. When combinatorial chemistry replaces traditional chemical techniques, laboratory design is dramatically different.

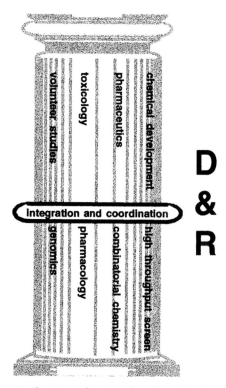

Figure 6.2   *Single site architectural analogy for drug R&D*

When new drugs are sought from molecular biological investigation, the personnel and the laboratory areas need to be changed. Increasingly, new technology has therefore been sought external to this infrastructure: the partnerships that have formed between small technology providers and larger companies are linked in much the same way as the pier buttresses are linked to the main body of a gothic cathedral via the flying buttress. This analogy is apposite for a number of reasons.

The architectural basis for the pier and flying buttress combination was to support the main structure and allow the construction of cathedrals to greater heights, where problems with wind were substantially increased. This had to be done with a minimum of stone on the outside of the building, to enlarge the windows, admit more light and generally to magnify the space inside to create a more impressive space in which to worship. In order to achieve these aims, additional force from the outside was applied to prevent collapse. One could say that the collaboration of a large company with a technology provider in a research project, or of a CRO to provide a part of the development work, buttresses the in-house efforts of the large company. If so, the downsizing of the past few years has left a structure within the large company that is not self-sustaining; the support of the partnership is required for it to attain the height to which it is built. Equally, the buttress cannot be left without a large company to support, for it too will collapse.

In the process of building cathedrals to this design, a great deal of trial and error was necessary to find the correct amount of buttressing that was necessary for structural integrity. There were of course failures, and in the absence of the sophistication of modern day architectural calculations, the communication of these collapses led to a rather empirical approach to cathedral design, in which errors were made on the safe side. A recent interpretation[85] is that some of the more flamboyant flying buttresses of the French school were overbuilt with safety in mind, and not therefore in the most efficient fashion: some of the buttresses were in fact made larger than was strictly necessary for the structural assistance needed to keep the cathedral from falling down. Does this suggest that as partnerships in the industry are becoming a more common approach, we still need to struggle to find the most efficient relative weighting between intra- and extramural resources, and the ways in which they best work together? Moreover, does it suggest that we will only learn the limits of what can be achieved from failed projects?

Although the current economic climate is in favour of small entrepreneurial ventures, the wise investor will remember 1991–2, when the situation rapidly changed for the worse (see p. 65). The prospects for the current generation are improved by the increasing emphasis on partnership and alliances that offer support to fledgling companies. Current advocates of partnership-based pharmaceutical R&D suggest that the fully integrated pharmaceutical company (FIPCO) is now permanently outdated. This is a recent development, certainly one that was not in place in 1991–2. In 1995, the funding of the biotechnology sector reached $3.6bn through alliances, over twice that of 1994, and equivalent to around 10% of total pharmaceutical R&D spending; at the same time the relative inflow of funds from acquisitions practically halved during the same period. Although two years' figures cannot constitute a definite trend, they do lend support to the suggestion that the flexibility of the alliance structure is regarded with increasing merit relative to the importance of acquisitions.

The question arises whether the stability of a large pharmaceutical company is required for such partnerships to work properly, or whether their co-ordinating role can be supplanted by yet another

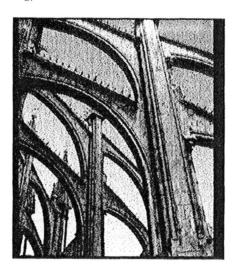

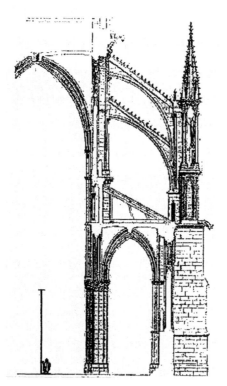

Figure 6.3   *Flying buttresses of Rheims Cathedral and the drawings of Viollet-le-Duc showing the cross-section and the structural action of the buttress; from Dictionnaire Raisonné de l'Architecture Française, vol. II, Paris*

small company. We have already seen the merger of ChemGenics with PerSeptive Biosystems, above. There are an increasing number of examples of partnerships between small companies that avoid the multinationals entirely. That between Sequana and Aurora Biosciences involving combinatorial chemistry and fluorescence-based high-throughput screening was referred to earlier (see section 5.2.1.2); Incyte has agreed with Affymetrix (a subsidiary of Affymax) to use the latter's technology to generate gene hybridisation expression data and with Scriptgen to provide data on bacterial function; T Cell Sciences has formed two alliances with a combinatorial partner (ArQule) and a provider of libraries of fermentation extracts (MYCOsearch), which can be fed into T Cell's screening and functional assays. ArQule has also agreed to collaborate on the development of ion channel modulators with another small company, ICAgen, and has acquired rights to methods for synthesis from Yale University. Also in the academic arena, Brandeis University has begun a project to discover peptidomimetics for anti-coagulation and fungal diseases with ArQule. The relationships between multiple small companies are becoming rapidly more complex: we need a structure by which it can be analysed.

Returning to the architectural analogy, beyond the buttressing of cathedrals, with time we can see that alternative designs were found to be even more effective for the construction of tall buildings. In the last century, the skyscrapers of Chicago were built with the benefits of new materials with an improved strength to weight ratio, and were the first to use the box-girder steel framework based on horizontal and vertical steel components, which could then be faced with brick.

Under this analogy, the process of preclinical pharmaceutical R&D is representable by the structure shown in Figure 6.4. The horizontal elements of integration and co-ordination connect the technology providers, represented by the vertical elements, and are an important component of this structure. In architectural terms, they are essential for structural integrity. The structure shown in Figure 6.4 has a number of advantages over the monolithic column construct of Figure 6.2, and may represent a means by which a network of entirely small companies can effectively perform drug R&D. Although the structure is suggestive of permanency, one needs to realise that as time proceeds, the components of the framework will change. Alliances are often designed to operate for only a portion of the drug development process. Some partners will fall away from the project, and others will need to be brought in at a later stage.

It is light for its height; the thin columns of the frame represent specific technologies essential for the project to succeed, provided by

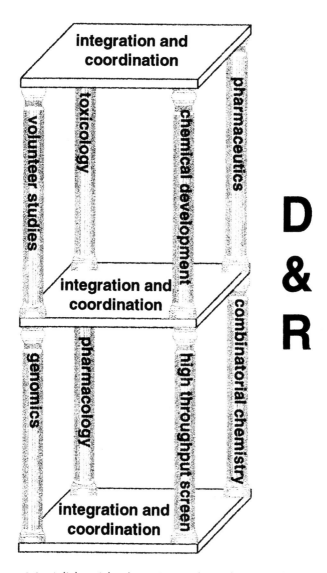

Figure 6.4   *A lightweight alternative to classical R&D architecture*

single discipline providers. Many of the peripheral elements which are embedded inflexibly in the single-column, large-company format, and represent the substantial overheads of that format, are either unrepresented, or brought in as needed. The sum total of these peripheral elements is a significant component of the resources in a large company, as was pointed out in section 2.4.1; however, they can be limiting to the flexibility of the organisation to adapt to new circumstances.

It is flexible; the pillars of specific disciplines of research and development are but examples of what may be needed to compose a total project. These may be increased or curtailed depending on the nature of the project at hand, and on the temporal stage of development of the project. A good example of a group of collaborators involving a combination of providers of technology for combinatorial synthesis, automated screening methodology and biochemistry/ pharmacology was that of Tripos, The Automation Partnership and the Cruciform Project described on p. 147.

The main purpose of this analogy is to enable the conceptual difference between the technology provider and the virtual company to be grasped. It also clarifies the difference between the technology provider and the multidisciplinary research project partner, which can be considered as providing a complete stage in the vertical development of the total R&D construct. It can be seen that the purposes of the CRO, the academic research group or the small entrepreneur are identical, although the ability of each to fit into the framework depends on the size and shape of the column that is required. The CRO's role may be to conduct an overflow project or to be a key provider of a number of services. Their experience of many different kinds of development projects has given them a breadth which few other companies in the pharmaceutical arena can match. Most of the virtual companies described below, particularly those which aim to carry a project through late development, use CROs extensively, if not exclusively, for the work they need to conduct. On the other hand, companies that are involved earlier in the drug discovery process can often also include providers from academia and the biotechnology sector.

To be fair, the disadvantages of this arrangement need to be understood too. One must ask what happens if one of the technology providers fails financially. Is the structure sufficiently robust to cope with the withdrawal of a vertical support, or will it collapse like a house of cards? Under these strains, the outcome depends critically on the strength of the horizontal layers, which must bear the burden of a weakened structure until a repair can be made, such as in the form of a new partner.

A major difference between the two structures of Figure 6.2 and Figure 6.4 is the increased emphasis on integration and co-ordination. The horizontal components of the latter are essential for the organisation of the research effort. The difficulty of organising this network in a successful manner should not be underestimated. Although these components have been represented as thin planes, in reality sufficient resources have to be placed in these horizontal components to facilitate the complex co-ordination of the project. Furthermore, their positioning at the top and the bottom of the technology columns is artistic licence. In reality, co-ordination needs to occur throughout the discovery and development process, in a continuous rather than discrete fashion.

The structure of Figure 6.4 places much emphasis on the integrative processes, in an effort to achieve more with less. This is not unlike the adaptive changes to structure which accompany the ageing of the human brain. Increasing integration becomes a compensatory mechanism for the decline in numbers of functional nerve cells which affect us all from our 20s onwards. Greater numbers of synapses enable people to maintain their mental faculties for many years of falling nerve cell numbers, because they can use their remaining resources more effectively.

6.3   TIME

Making partnerships work is not a trivial exercise.[86] Each side can rationally believe it is getting less of an advantage than it is due. For a start, despite all the talk of the advantages of flexibility brought by collaborative enterprises, a successful partnership cannot be built in a rush. Establishing the first piece of work in a collaborative partnership with an external body almost always takes longer than conducting the same piece of work in-house. This is not a property of the collaboration *per se*, but a factor that is related to the arrangements that need to be in place before the co-operative working relationship can begin. Negotiations between one company and a number of potential partners often take place in parallel, at least part of the way. Beyond identification of the possibilities, secrecy agreements have to be agreed, the terms discussed and a contract secured. Facets of such contracts are mentioned below.

A project that is heavily reliant on collaborations can be substantially delayed by these setting-up periods unless a great deal of foresight is practised. An alternative method is to set up a loose network of collaborators as a prime initial step. Once these are in place, they may be used as needed in an *ad hoc* fashion to fulfil the various multidisciplinary tasks that are necessary in the project. The network may be changed with time as new features are required, or alternative collaborators need to be brought in to complement or replace existing ones.

The value of the working relationships that are established between partners improves with time. The main feature is trust; initial contact is formal and progress based on agreements made in writing. As time develops, decisions and action can be taken on a less formal basis, by verbal means. In addition to human understanding, linked procedures and other efficiencies (such as familiarity with the technology of the project) also develop with time, and the full benefits accrue slowly.

Time can be a great frustration in developing relationships, especially in long-distance partnerships when the overlap in working hours is a fraction of the normal working day (see section 3.7). Naturally, with distance a factor, the communications between both sides will normally permit fewer face-to-face meetings than is possible in a larger single company. Communications as a whole are a central element to any successful relationship.

6.4 COMMUNICATION CHANNELS

For an organisation which wishes to use extramural studies widely, getting a group of collaborators to work together in a network involves more than merely communication via a central point. A network of collaborators remains, to date, a model which has an insubstantial track record. It represents a great challenge as a means of conducting pharmaceutical research and development. Interest in this model is intense because it offers a dramatic change to the historic *modus operandi* of the industry.

First, and most importantly, the modes—rather than the media—of communication. If the network can be conceived of as a web, then communication must be possible around the periphery as well as via the centre. The extramural participants must be aware of the existence and broad operation of the other participants. The contact points within this web need to be defined and identified to everybody. These people within their various organisations need sufficient seniority to act with authority, without undue reference to their line management, which can cause confusion and delay. Personalities need to be able to work together, and individuals who are good communicators are essential. Shy scientists, happier with test tubes than telephones, need not apply. In this respect, team building amongst the key points of contact within the web is highly relevant.

Despite tangential communication around the web's periphery, it is along radial routes that planning of the project is conducted. The central administrative function is crucial in overviewing the project management, setting the work to be done, the time by which it must be done and the resources that need to be allocated. Setting deadlines and plans that are solid and which do not continually change is important for the stability of the operation, and keeping contractors focused on the tasks at hand. The flexibility of a project that incorporates multiple collaborators can collapse into instability if the organisation is not clear and well respected.

The omnipotent requirements of a project manager have been emphasised in section 3.8. For management of a multiple-collaborative project, this requirement is magnified, since the anticipation of problems becomes a vital means of avoiding them. Project planning is a bigger issue with so much work being conducted extramurally. Sufficient attention to detail is necessary, and understanding of all the component parts of the project plan is needed in order that it can work.[87] It is all too easy to forget that one small piece of the work that needs to be conducted, on the false assumption that it falls within one collaborator's field of involvement, when in fact the said collaborator is unaware of this requirement.

6.5   COMMUNICATION METHODS

Single-site projects operate substantially through decisions made at meetings, where all the disciplines and people involved in the project may be represented. This is not possible with distantly separated groups, where the bulk of communication will be by telephony, and communications are a much more important element. Where interaction is necessary between two or more extramural groups, it helps greatly to have had face-to-face meetings early on in the collaboration, but this is not usually feasible on a regular basis. Certainly, arranging project meetings of multiple components of the type common in large pharmaceutical companies is next to impossible.

The improvements in electronic communication over the past 10 years are of dramatic importance to the feasibility of collaborative work in general, although the changes in the next 10 are likely to be even more dramatic. There has been a great change in our concept of the world: both geographically, and in terms of time. Distance is no longer a significant impediment. Both cultural and technological factors underpin this change. Culturally, business by telephone is increasingly common and people recognise the need to reach out and be reached by this medium; the use and acceptance of portable phones is rapidly increasing. The need for personal contact is diminishing in all areas of business because it is less time-efficient. In terms of technology, we have seen how the relatively old and simple technology of the fax machine has enabled huge increases in the rapidity of transfer of data. It is indicative of the pace of change that, while the impact of fax technology is still not fully developed, its replacement by computer-controlled scanning and digitisation technology can be foreseen. Fax technology is very strong in its capacity to communicate simultaneously to groups of people and in the communication of written documents. Its formality lends a degree of comfort to parties that have yet to develop a relationship of trust. (Its counterpart in large organisations to facilitate interdepartmental communication was the written memorandum, now surpassed by company e-mail, of which more later.) Yet its immediacy can impart a drive and momentum to the collaboration as rapid as any single-site project.

The deficiencies of the fax can equally be seen from the tendency for telephonic communication in mature collaborative efforts (paralleled by the acceptance of verbal communication rather than memoranda in smooth-running, trusting companies). Communication that involves writing is inevitably slower than communication based solely on talking. The formality of the written form can lead to greater degrees of conservativeness. The written answer will normally be a conservative estimate. The verbal answer may also contain a range of possibilities, including some more optimistic estimates. Which answer is correct is, to a certain extent, unimportant: the verbal route has elicited more information, and therefore is more useful.

Information technology (IT) is a powerful tool with the potential to change fundamentally the way companies carry out research, and has great applicability to devolved projects. The pharmaceutical industry has been a major purchaser of computer technology, particularly to enhance its R&D function. The use of advanced data handling and robotic techniques has only been possible through the increased use of computerised technology. As far as information itself is concerned, IT is becoming increasingly used by the scientist at the bench. Primary literature references are still not usually directly available through the computer terminal, but the trend for electronic journals indicates that this will shortly become widespread. In the meantime, networked CD-ROM machines with journals in this format can provide an alternative method of delivering data to distant locations. This issue is of prime importance to delocalised bodies conducting research or development, since access to large libraries is often difficult outside an academic setting.

Electronic mail is a versatile means of maintaining communication within groups. This is especially valuable where communication is necessary between more than two participants in the project, since simultaneous communication can easily occur between 3, 4 or 20 groups. Electronic mail also offers the possibility of sending computer files of data between sites. This is conventionally done in large companies without difficulty because common software platforms are used. In a network of collaborators, the software may be partially compatible, or even completely incompatible. It may not be cost-effective to convert such data, depending on how much would need to be manually entered. This issue is particularly relevant for the compilation of regulatory submissions, such as IND or CTX documents.

There is an increasing body of work on the electronic document and data handling in the pharmaceutical industry. Three trends are evident:[88]

- compatibility issues are becoming less of a problem
- computer systems validation is becoming more relevant and difficult as systems become more complex
- the incursion of computer technology into the pharmaceutical industry is presenting many challenges regarding training and changes to operating procedures

The first two issues particularly affect the operation of work done in partnerships, where data need to flow between groups. Compatibility of computer systems is one problem that needs to be addressed if collaborators are to use electronic means for exchanging data effectively. This is most keenly seen in the moves to computerise submissions to regulatory authorities as CANDAs (computer-assisted new drug applications) and CAPLAs (computer-assisted product licence applications). There is an uncertainty about the eventual format of such applications,[88] which is leading to a lack of direction in other processes leading to the provision of regulatory submissions. At the preclinical end, key issues concerning compatibility of software programs are less of a problem than 10 years ago. The common business platform for most desktop applications is based on Microsoft Windows, except for a minority use of Macintosh systems in academia. Nevertheless, problems do still arise that limit the interchange of data between collaborators. These problems are usually not insurmountable, though they do lead to inefficiencies in the research and development process.

A network of collaborators would benefit greatly from the ability to append electronic contributions from participants to a central database or set of documents (e.g. for regulatory submission) with potential for immediate import of such data without the need for substantial manual intervention. This requires that each collaborator is able to submit such data in a compatible format (such as a spreadsheet for data or a word-processed document for written submissions) and that the central administrative function can handle such files in an efficient way. Electronic data can be manipulated by various editorial techniques to create documents or databases from diverse origins. Submission can be made across the Internet, and there is great potential for the use of this infrastructure in bringing disparate groups together. The advantages of intranets, which provide the capacity to communicate by methods similar to the World Wide Web, but within companies, suggest that building a similar secure environment for collaborating groups would have significant advantages. The term 'collaboratory' is entering our language to describe this type of activity, in which research findings can be posted to a common notice-board and viewed by other parties with granted access rights as soon as they are available. Issues of security are particularly important for this kind of venture in the pharmaceutical industry, and there is substantial research going on towards the enablement of secure links via the Internet. Newer encryption methods have application in other industrial sectors, particularly banking, and it seems certain that technology to address this issue will be available in a short time. Quintiles have invested heavily in computerised acquisition of data, and the construction of a $70–80m Wide Area Network, with great benefit to multisite clinical studies, each contributing data that need to be amalgamated at a central location; clearly, there is great potential for the utility of this type of data manipulation in preclinical as well as clinical investigation. The benefit of this real-time updating mechanism can be substantial when regulatory submissions are required.

The argument for setting up more elaborate means of communication such as video conference links may be apparent, but as it normally involves installation of specialised telephone lines it is beneficial only with long-term partners for whom regular visual contact is essential. However, a substantial amount of work is currently taking place in the telecommunications industry that may revolutionise the ways we can communicate in the future. Developments in data compression technology can allow faster transfer of large amounts of information, such as televisual images, down an ordinary copper phone line. The computer chip manufacturer Intel has announced its intention to install videophone capability onto its future Pentium-based personal computers. These advances are sure to permit great flexibility in communication methods, with many concomitant advantages relative to those that require installation of high bandwidth telephone lines. Computer technology will underpin the communications between partners in a much more extensive (and invasive) way than is currently normal. Harmonious, secure and fast electronic communication is undoubtedly the future for networked groups of collaborators, with great possibilities for transfer of text, image, data and voice by means that ignore distance.

Location, despite the advances in communications, is an additional determinant factor in some collaborations. There is a substantial group of small companies that has formed around Boston in the US. A recent study of the biotechnology industry in this area showed that 35% of companies felt that close proximity to leading university and medical research sites was paramount.[89] One reason for this was, presumably, access to good libraries; another, perhaps, that access to the latest scientific data, and to the leaders in the field was better. However, geographical propinquity is not all that it seems. Academic experts spend as much time away from their lab as in it; real access to the latest developments is through personal contacts (such as encounters at the right scientific meetings) that may be quite feasible between scientific groups who are based long distances apart.

One tangible factor to consider in any drug research project is that physical movements of drug samples need to occur. In this respect, but also in general within the project, foresight is essential. Even the best laid plans do not always proceed smoothly: packages are delayed, lost in customs, mislaid in the internal mail, buried under another despatch at the outgoing end. Lack of foresight is a disaster in terms of ensuring sufficient material is at the correct site at the correct time. Keeping track of what was sent to whom, when, how much sample was used and when additional quantities will be necessary is highly complicated. This is less of a problem when dealing with one development compound than when dealing with thousands of candidate compounds in research. However, even in the former case the number of linked studies is greater and problems with scheduling are still often apparent.

6.6　SETTING UP A CONTRACT

Much has been written about setting up contracts to establish the ground rules for collaborative efforts. There is no such thing as a standard contract; it depends on the type of work. Konecny[61] listed twelve components of a model contract which have been drawn up from experience and joint work by government-sponsored industrial/ academic conferences:

- concise statement of goals and schedule for achieving them
- assignment of responsibility for various parts of the work
- meetings and reports—when and how
- protection of information, by principal investigator and other workers
- ownership of intellectual property, royalties
- exclusivity—preventing partner working in the same or similar field for competitors
- publication procedure
- remuneration and expenses
- revision of the contract
- duration of contract
- arbitration and governing law
- liability of sponsor in the event of consequences of academic investigator's actions

The problem with regard to academic collaborations concerning publication was dealt with in section 3.5. An added element of complexity is brought about by the increasing requirement of academic institutions for royalties on work associated with commercially rewarding projects. Partly as a result of the increasing commercialism in the academic sector, it is now well recognised that confidentiality is preserved while patents are filed. With regard to strategic partnerships with small biotechnology companies, the issue of ownership of rights and royalty payments is a major component of the deal. This is not the case with straight contract work with CROs, although some such organisations occasionally like to see consultancy agreements in place in recognition of the intellectual involvement with the sponsored work, if that pertains.

An imaginative solution to the problem of patent rights is to be found in the 1996 agreement between Peptide Therapeutics (PT) and Alizyme (AL) for combinatorial chemistry (Figure 6.5). The central issue was the need for the providers (PT) to retain majority rights to the libraries of compounds, and for the buyer (AL) to acquire majority rights to the lead compounds from the libraries that it wished to develop. In Figure 6.5, the royalty percentage x is substantially less than 50. The balance between these competing priorities is nicely made by the provision for the provider to acquire

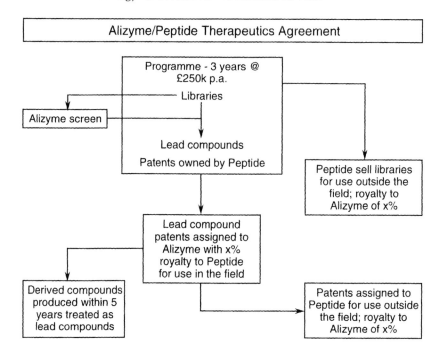

Figure 6.5   *Intellectual property agreement between Peptide Therapeutics and Alizyme*

reciprocal rights for the lead compounds in areas outside the buyer's therapeutic interests.

A key component of any arrangement that is struck is flexibility; inevitably, the best laid plans do not always unfold as expected, and it is important that such upsets do not impair the ability of the partnership to change tack (subject to the wish of both parties to so continue). Some of the companies referred to below, such as KS Biomedix, operate in areas of early research that are difficult to plan over the lifetime of a collaboration. Their philosophy is to rely more on trust and understanding as a result of relationships that have built up over many years, rather than to set up formal contracts.

6.7   CASE HISTORIES

There are a number of small companies that have been set up with the express purpose of conducting drug research or development in a delocalised sense. The vogue adjective for their style of operation is virtual since they perform little or no actual practical scientific work.

Their business is based around project management, in the research or the developmental sense. They use a combination of partners, from CROs to academic groups, or work with small companies in the biotechnology sector. Some of these companies have been extensively involved in collaborations more by accident than design. This is not to say that the reasons for them operating this way were not apparent at the outset. Rather, it is to point out the difference between those who entered this realm with open eyes and a belief that it would be successful, and those who pursued the path by reason of necessity rather than strategy.

6.7.1 By design

6.7.1.1 *Vanguard Medica*

Vanguard Medica was set up in 1992 by Sir John Vane and Professor Eric Änggård, together with a number of doyens of the pharmaceutical industry, from both the UK and the US, such as Dr Roger Brimblecombe, Dr Bill Duncan and Dr Chuck Smith. Through Sir John Vane, they have contact with the academic William Harvey Research Institute. They are flexible in their aims, having a number of projects in collaboration with larger pharmaceutical companies as well as their own projects. Initial funding was provided by venture capitalists, which initially raised £6m, and later raised a further £11.2m. In May 1996, the company was floated on the UK stock market, raising a further £30m, capitalising the company at £140m. Vanguard is building a portfolio of compounds through licensing and collaborative agreements. The earliest it expects products to reach the market is in 2000 or 2001.

An example is the development of Lilly's LTB_4 antagonist, LY293111, for diseases with an inflammatory component, which Vanguard took over from Lilly at the end of Phase I. Among the many potential applications, including inflammatory bowel disease, asthma and arthritis, Vanguard have focused on psoriasis, an indication that they are also pursuing with a natural plant extract licensed from the Strathclyde Institute for Drug Research. They are also pursuing collaborations with British Technology Group for a compound for hyperphosphataemia in renal failure which is currently in Phase I development; and with a $5HT_{1D}$ partial agonist from SmithKline Beecham for the treatment of migraine, which was also taken over early on. This is an example of a compound for which SmithKline Beecham accorded low priority in development. Vanguard's role is therefore partly to cater for the less worthy candidates which swell a

Table 6.3   Compounds undergoing development by Vanguard Medica

Compound	Collaborator	Therapy	Stage
VML 251	SB	Migraine	Phase III
VML 252	BTG and King's College, London	Hyperphosphataemia	Phase I
VML 295	Lilly	Psoriasis	Phase IIa
		Inflammatory Bowel Disease	Preclinical
VML 262	Strathclyde University (Strathclyde Institute for Drug Research)	Psoriasis (topical)	Preclinical
VML 275	UCL (University College London)	UVA and UVB protection	Preclinical

company's development pipelines beyond their in-house capability. The indications are that this type of opportunity will occur more frequently as large companies run their internal resources in an increasingly lean fashion. This deal is also interesting because of the way both the risk and the reward of the project are shared between the two sides. Vanguard is paid for achieving clinical milestones, as well as in terms of a share of the future net operating receipts, and is allocated co-promotion rights for the US market. Vanguard is therefore proposing to take this compound through the entire development process alone, a potentially risky venture but one that will bring substantial rewards if successful. In total, there are five collaborative arrangements on compounds in development with major pharmaceutical companies and academic institutes (see Table 6.3). They use CROs predominantly to conduct the necessary work, and consultants extensively in areas where they believe they need help, for instance chemical development.

6.7.1.2   Triangle

Triangle was set up by a number of senior executives from the Wellcome Research Centre in North Carolina after the closure of this site following the take-over by Glaxo in 1995. Its CEO, the former Wellcome head of R&D, Dr David Barry, has maintained his therapeutic focus (virology) at Wellcome in the new venture, rapidly forming partnerships with a number of companies to develop four anti-HIV, one anti-cancer and one anti-herpes product. One of the collaborations is with Mitsubishi to develop their AIDS drug MKC-442, for which Triangle has an option to carry out development through Phase Ia and IIa human studies. Some of their development compounds come from Emory University and concern other drugs for HIV. The company contracts out nearly all of its work, but has limited laboratory facilities to conduct some applied studies, such as elucidation of the mode of action of in-licensed compounds. The company's aim is to add value by moving the compounds to the next stage of development, such as from preclinical to Phase I, after which it may look for other partners.

6.7.1.3 Alizyme

Alizyme was set up in 1995 by Dr Andrew Porter to concentrate on the early development of therapies for gastrointestinal diseases and obesity. The company immediately set about forming alliances with other small companies as technology providers. The partnership with Peptide Therapeutics in the area of combinatorial chemistry has been mentioned previously (section 6.6). In addition, it has chosen to work with Oxford Molecular for its rational drug design capabilities. Deal structure incorporates the normal elements of milestone payments and royalties on any products, in addition to research costs. Other agreements are in place with British Technology Group, Institute of Food Research, University of Strathclyde and Rowett Research Services.

The projects that Alizyme are investigating are either at a research or early developmental stage. They include investigation of novel inhibitors of pancreatic lipase and amylase which are involved in the digestion of fats, and are potentially useful in obesity. Diarrhoea, irritable bowel disease and gastrointestinal infections are also therapeutic targets in which Alizyme is interested. Following completion of early clinical trials (Phase II), the company will probably seek partners from the larger pharmaceutical companies for later development.

Alizyme's strategy is different from Vanguard Medica's in so far as the projects are earlier in development, and include research work. By focusing on gastrointestinal diseases, a category including obesity for which there is clearly a large market, the hurdle of bioavailability which is normally so critical for oral delivery may be bypassed. In fact candidates with poor absorption characteristics or high rates of first-pass metabolic transformations may actually be preferred because systemic exposure is minimised. This also opens the way for treatments based on larger molecules, such as some of the products of biotechnology, although the problems of proteolytic degradation in the stomach (prior to a desired site of action in the intestines) will still have to be dealt with.

6.7.1.4   KS Biomedix

This company was founded in 1990 using capital from a previous diagnostics venture, which was set up in 1986 by Dr Kim Tan, an émigré from British academia. The diagnostics venture was reasonably successful, for example selling kits for determination of morphine to the US Army, and for the diagnosis of disease in poultry. Thus, KS Biomedix was able to run with purely private finance until 1995, when it achieved a UK stock market listing. Partly because of the relative lack of need of financial investment, the company has been able to let the science speak for itself and does not bathe in the ultraviolet glare of press attention, more typical of some others in the biotechnology industry.

KS Biomedix (KSB) provides support for those academic projects it sees as having commercial application. The support is much more than purely financial investment, and KSB is actively involved with the management of the projects' intermediate development. Preclinical work, including toxicology, is subcontracted by KSB up to a proof-of-principle clinical trial in man. Beyond Phase II, KSB normally seeks to out-license, but the financial deal that it will seek will depend on the project and the partner. In this regard, KSB sees itself as a very flexible organisation.

In addition to Dr Tan, the company is advised by a board of eminent scientists with extensive industrial as well as academic experience of relevance for the therapeutic aims of the projects in hand. These are:

- Rheumatoid arthritis, low molecular weight compound, currently in Phase II. The approach employed is to modify the release of glucose-6-phosphate dehydrogenase, since this enzyme is increased fourfold in the human condition as well as in animal models.
- Osteoarthritis, low molecular weight compound, currently in Phase II. A synergistic combination of two known drugs inhibited development of disease in a mouse model of osteoarthritis; neither drug alone was effective.
- High affinity sheep monoclonal antibodies for use in oncology and haemostasis. Sheep monoclonal antibodies potentially have orders of magnitude of greater potency than their analogues in mice, and may bring about substantially enhanced selectivity such as in the targeting of chemotherapeutic agents for cancer*.

---

* Now licensed by Roche in an unspecified disease area.

A similar model of operation is displayed by Prolifix, which acts as a focal point for the co-ordination of the activities of around 60 academic scientists spread throughout Europe. Their research is directed towards drugs for control of cellular proliferation, with particular expertise in the area of high-throughput screening. A deal was struck in 1995 with Chugai.[90]

6.7.1.5 Fieldcastle

Fieldcastle Inc. was set up by Dr Hank Agersborg, formerly Research President of Wyeth-Ayerst, with the concept of fully outsourcing the development of pharmaceuticals, via the setting up of multiple companies, each concerned with the development of an individual drug. These fully outsourced companies have been given the acronym FOSCOs. According to Agersborg, the central problem in pharmaceutical development is the cost, and this applies for the newly founded biotechnology companies as much as for the larger multinationals. Typically, small companies which are set up with venture capital backing will require a total of over $100m, sometimes up to twice that, before any return is made. Despite a substantial initial venture capital investment, by the time any return can be made it will have become greatly diluted by additional investment from share offerings, and the eventual returns can be expected to be modest.

The FOSCO model aims to pare development costs to the bone in an attempt to achieve Phase III results with as little as $10m, and to allow the venture capital company to own 50% of the FOSCO following the institutional public offering (IPO). It is recognised that not all drug development is successful, but that when it does work, returns can be high when a product reaches the market. FOSCOs are a possibility in today's environment because of the large service community of CROs and other external bodies that can facilitate drug development.

Minimal infrastructure costs are an essential component of the FOSCO's strength. There are no laboratory facilities, and very low running costs due to the skeletal staffing of the organisation. Multiple development of more than one drug can share resources of coordinators, but the legal company entities are separate. Delayed studies and slippage result in alterations in timing of funding requirements, but not in additional costs associated with maintaining a large in-house team.

Unlike many of the other small virtual companies, FOSCOs entertain the possibility of retaining marketing rights in core areas and/or territories. The effect of this strategy is to maximise the worth of the

Table 6.4   *Drug development costs using the FOSCO model*

Stage	Costs ($m)	Probability of success per stage[a]	Expected cost per stage ($m)
Preclinical	0.75	0.75	1
Phase I/IIA	1.25	0.5	2.5
Phase IIB	2.0	0.5	4.0
Phase III	6.0	0.6	10.0
Administration[b]	4.7	0.85	5.1
Total	14.7		22.6

[a] Figures estimated from Table 1.5, Recombinant Capital column.
[b] Burn rate calculated as $0.3m per year during development, and $1.0m per year through NDA; development time 9 years and 2 years NDA.

company that is successful in taking a product to market. The FOSCO is designed to grow substantially when a product reaches the market, and an IPO would be scheduled to precede product launch. Prior to that, company value increases with clinical evidence for utility of the product; and decreases to zero if the product fails during clinical investigation.

As yet, success has not been demonstrated in a commercial sense. The most advanced project currently under investigation is by a company called CollaGenex. Their product, which has an indication for periodontitis originated at Johnson and Johnson and has completed Phase III clinical trials and an NDA filing, for a total cost of less than $6m. The work was conducted at a number of well-established CROs. Other projects are in early development and include a neuron-desensitising drug for diabetic neuropathy, rhinitis and incontinence; and a natural peptide active in healing that is being investigated for burn treatment. Regarding CollaGenex, following the NDA filing with the FDA, an IPO has been undertaken. The original investors owned about half the company following the IPO. Agersborg estimates the drug development costs employing the FOSCO model are as shown in Table 6.4 for a generalised acute therapy, and have been adhered to in the case of CollaGenex.

For those who are familiar with the estimates for drug development costs estimated by Grabowski[29] or by the Lehman Brothers' report in 1996[32] (see Tables 1.5 and 1.6) the absolute estimate of $14.7m is almost incredible in its modesty; even when taking into account the fact that each of these figures needs to be divided by the probability of success in each stage in order to reach the expected costs of successful launch, the eventual sum, at $22.6m, is still a fraction of previous estimates (Table 1.5). Agersborg even argues that the probabilities of success historically evident from data from large pharmaceutical companies—such as from Wenzel (Table 1.5)—can be bettered with carefully selected clinical targets and drug candidates. This would reduce the figures in Table 6.4 even further. If this model does succeed in bringing pharmaceutical products to market for such limited financial outlay, the future for the industry is surely bright; and the future for Fieldcastle brilliant.

FOSCOs are different from some of the other virtual companies mentioned here in working exclusively by contract rather than by partnership. As mentioned earlier, the major difference between these two modes of outsourcing relates to the division of intellectual property rights. In many relationships, the solution to this problem can be an unwieldy one. However, the use of contracts in a research sense poses difficulties if inventiveness is sought from the contractor, because no rights to the invention are on offer. FOSCOs are likely to work best where straight development is required, without any research element. The expertise necessary for late-stage development includes a greater emphasis on regulatory considerations than in other examples of virtual companies. In addition, the FOSCO is happy with the concept of taking a product all the way through to market, and beyond, whereas most of the other virtual companies are keen to find partners for late development. The final difference between the FOSCO model and others is that because each project is handled by a separate legal entity, it is wound up if the clinical trials are unsuccessful. Resources, office space and personnel are shared between different companies, but from the viewpoint of the investor, the financial backing is focused on one project. Naturally, this offers a significant up-side if the project is successful as well as a significant, but contained, down-side if it is not.

6.7.1.6   AMRAD

AMRAD was established in 1988 with seed capital from the Victorian state government of Australia to commercialise the science of the Melbourne research institutes. Now a public listed company, it is 35% Victorian government owned, with other pharmaceutical companies such as MSD (Australia) also retaining significant shareholdings.

It has extensive collaborations with 11 research institutes through-out Australia on which it has first rights for any inventions which derive therefrom, and in return these institutes maintain a total 10% share interest in AMRAD. The AMRAD model is interesting because in addition to the network of academic collaborators for the research which is anticipated to provide the long-term future, the company maintains a marketing arm which supplies the day-to-day funding upon which it is based. Thus, AMRAD has co-marketing agreements with major pharmaceutical companies for commonly prescribed drugs such as simvastatin (cholesterol-lowering) and acyclovir (antiviral). This allows the Australian physician an option with a larger indigenous component and has produced a rapid increase in sales volume, from Aus$0.3m to Aus$75m from 1988 to 1996.

Besides the commercial arm, the research pipeline has a number of components, the most advanced of which is a vaccine for rotavirus, which is a principal cause of gastroenteritis in young children, both in Australia and in the third world. AMRAD is seeking partners for development at an early stage. There are a number of other projects at a research or preclinical stage, from antivirals for hepatitis B to vaccines or other approaches to HIV. The HIV projects are based on the observation that progression from HIV-positivity to AIDS does not seem to occur in patients whose HIV strain is defective in a certain gene, called *nef.* Inhibition of the *nef* gene or inoculation with a *nef*-deficient HIV strain itself may offer potential approaches to the disease.

AMRAD has a specific advantage from its location in terms of access to natural products, and has developed a substantial collection of samples from plants and fungi from Australia. It has come to an agreement with neighbouring Borneo for access to its biota, and similarly with Antarctica. In order to screen these samples, AMRAD has a five-year collaboration with Panlabs, from which it has gained immediate access to external expertise it did not possess, and meanwhile it has slowly built up an in-house capability. From these efforts, the subsidiary AMRAD National Products has arisen, which has formed a collaboration with Chugai.

AMRAD's success seems to have been built upon a niche strategy that plays to the strengths of its geographical location and national pharmaceutical market. It has harnessed the efforts of the national academic community and looked to collaborative expertise to progress projects in disciplines or techniques where it was weak. In other areas, it has sought in-licensing deals for new products that it felt it could improve upon, and will seek out-licensing deals to progress its products through late-stage development. Overall, the company bears similarities to KS Biomedix, but also includes a marketing function which provides a financial stream to finance its research efforts.

6.7.2 By necessity

6.7.2.1 *Napp/Mundipharma/Purdue Pharma*

Napp in the UK is one of a number of companies that form part of a privately held collection under common ownership of the Sackler

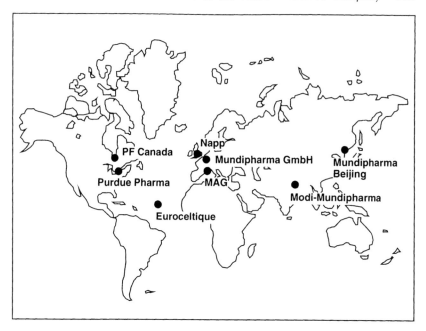

Figure 6.6   *Companies owned by the Sackler family world-wide*

family. Others in a similar position include Purdue Frederick and Purdue Pharma in the US, a separate Purdue Frederick in Canada, and Mundipharma GmbH in Germany and Mundipharma AG in Switzerland. Patents are assigned to Euroceltique SA, a Luxembourg company. There are additional smaller companies in Israel, India and China which are also under individual local management. Though under common private ownership, they have their own local management and operate largely independently of one another (see Figure 6.6). Their business focus is in developing and selling controlled release versions of existing drugs such as morphine and theophylline.

The local companies have hitherto seen advantage in operating independently because they can respond more accurately and quickly to market conditions in their home territory. However, in a desire to undertake a bigger project involving substantial commitment to fundamental research, towards a new chemical entity, commonality of purpose has been recognised as essential. Towards this end, the International Molecular Discovery group has functioned across local company divisions and through an extensive network of collaborative ventures with both industrial and academic partners. The goal of the first project set up in 1993 to discover an inhibitor of phosphodiesterase 4 for the treatment of asthma has been pursued through a number

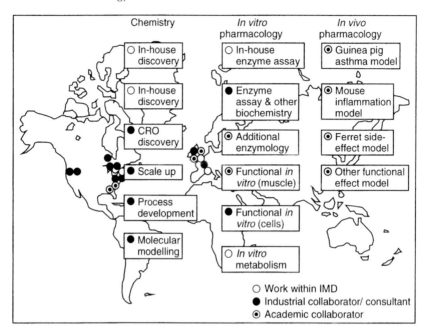

Figure 6.7 *Organisation by location of International Molecular Discovery*

of laboratories world-wide, as shown in Figure 6.7. The concept of PDE4 inhibition is that a selective drug with this property would have both bronchodilatory and anti-inflammatory effects in asthma, but without some of the cardiovascular and other side-effects with which a non-selective PDE inhibitor such as theophylline is burdened. Through its collaborations, the group has been able to tap into first-class expertise in the field of asthma from a variety of backgrounds without the time delay and difficulty associated with building such an expertise in-house. This is very much in line with the original concept of the virtual corporation from Jan Hopkins, the DEC executive who described it as 'an enterprise that can marshal more resources than it currently has on its own, using collaborations from both inside and outside its business'.[91] Consultancy advice, such as in molecular modelling, is an important component of this project. Although there has been discovery chemistry work carried out in both Napp and Mundipharma AG, until very recently there has been no practical biology to screen or subsequently to test candidate compounds. The crux of this organisation is multidisciplinary fore-sight and early planning to cope with problems before they arise. The time taken to source component parts of the project externally has been cited earlier (see section 3.6) as a potential delay for outsourced projects, but if addressed early this disadvantage can be minimised. A substantial degree of logistical organisation has been necessary in order to set up systems of testing that enable rapid feedback of results to the medicinal chemist. This system has not been without its problems. However, it would not have been possible for such a group to successfully bring a compound into Phase I volunteer trials (as it has done) without this unconventional (but increasingly modern) approach.

The advantages of flexibility that accrue from outsourcing are particularly evident for smaller enterprises. The risk they take in committing their future to a particular strategy is reduced if that strategy is played out through collaborative ventures. This is particularly so for the small company wishing to undertake research into new chemical entities. Napp, along with Mundipharma and Purdue Pharma, have pursued the collaborative route because the alternative would have placed the companies' futures in jeopardy should the project fail to be commercially rewarding. The success or otherwise of this exercise is not yet established in this regard, but it is a novel approach, which others may follow.

6.7.2.2   Xenova

Xenova was established in 1987 by Dr Louis Nisbet, a microbiologist with previous experience at Smith Kline & French (now SmithKline Beecham). It has established its reputation as a research-based biotechnology company with a proprietary screening technology (known as ASSET, advanced screening technology) and a unique collection of fungal, bacterial and plant organisms from which it can provide leads for a variety of projects. Its therapeutic focus has been on cancer, immune disorders and viral diseases. Over the years it has formed alliances and collaborations with a number of companies, such as DuPont, Organon, Suntory, Genentech, Roche, Genzyme, Pharma-Genics and Warner-Lambert. Its alliance with Suntory has existed since 1993, and was recently renewed until 1997; several milestone payments have been made in regard to this collaboration, which concerns small molecule drugs for the treatment of immuno-inflammatory diseases such as rheumatoid arthritis. In addition, Xenova retains its proprietary compounds, including a compound for multidrug resistance, and a plasminogen activator inhibitor for thrombosis which are in Phase I. However, the British start-up company has not enjoyed unalloyed success recently. Its collaboration with Roche, involving the preclinical investigation of a T cell inhibitor for non-asthma-related allergic indications and organ transplant rejection, was suspended in 1995. In order to adapt to difficult financial circumstances, it has gone through two further rounds of fundraising and has enforced substantial redundancies over the last 18 months or so; it is increasing its emphasis on becoming a decentralised drug discovery and development company rather than just a technology provider. This is most obviously represented in the collaboration with the Cancer Research Campaign, which involves development of a novel anti-cancer lead and related series of compounds. A question arises whether Xenova finds itself as a frequently cited 'virtual research' company by design or accident. Although it has been included in the 'by necessity' bracket, its current strategic involvement with virtuality seems to be representative of only one of multiple strands. Xenova's future development could proceed along the more traditional lines of a research provider, or it could expand its virtual development capabilities; time will tell.*

6.7.2.3   EuroAlliance

EuroAlliance is a consortium of four small European pharmaceutical companies, Alfa Schiapparelli Wasserman (Italy), Lafon (France), Lacer (Spain) and Merckle (Germany). It has been announced recently that EuroAlliance has completed a Phase I trial with a novel anti-inflammatory, ML3000. Phase II trials are expected to commence at the end of 1996. This compound is reported to possess fewer side-effects than other NSAIDs, since it combines cyclooxygenase and 5-lipoxygenase inhibition. The production of inflammatory leukotrienes is thought by some to be increased as a result of inhibition of cyclooxygenase, and this can be attenuated by the concomitant inhibition of 5-lipoxygenase. ML3000 was originally discovered by Merckle, but is being developed by EuroAlliance for the primary indication of rheumatism, with potential utility as an anti-asthmatic, antipyretic and analgesic.

As this is a combination of small companies, it is clear that the strategic reasons for co-operation are based on producing an organisation with sufficient resources to enter into the new chemical entity research arena. However, the mechanisms for the operation of the alliance are unclear. It would seem that success is best assured in this venture if direction and decision making are centralised rather than dispersed. There is a danger that the ability to make rapid progress can be impeded by the need to resort to committee procedures.

---

* Following this prediction, Xenova has recently announced the formation of a discovery division called MetaXen, to include its preclinical researchers, in partnership with Arris Pharmaceuticals. The remainder of Xenova will presumably more clearly align itself into the 'virtual' model.

The main disadvantage of drug R&D by a consortium of companies is that each can exert its own independent choices regarding when and whether to take the next step during the development of the project. Differences of scientific opinion are one thing, but of more concern is the potential withdrawal of a partner for purely financial reasons that have nothing whatsoever to do with the project at hand. The principles of project management are used in drug R&D precisely to harmonise the different priorities that may compete amongst different departments within a single organisation. At the heart of project management is a project manager. An alliance of independent companies poses significant challenges since there is not going to be a leader unless all of the partners except one abdicate their prerogative for self-determination. Leadership by committee has a tendency to lead to delay and lack direction, in the absence of such abdication*.

6.7.2.4 Shire Pharmaceuticals

Shire Pharmaceuticals in the UK bears many similarities to Fieldcastle (section 6.7.1.5). This company was set up in 1986 and has projects spanning the spectrum of pharmaceutical development, from pre-clinical to marketing. It has a therapeutic focus on metabolic bone diseases, and on CNS disorders such as Alzheimer's. Shire's pre-clinical projects include bisphosphonates and phosphate binders for osteoporosis, utilising oral and transdermal delivery systems. It has a major product in development for Alzheimer's disease, galanthamine, which is a cholinesterase inhibitor that is more specific and less toxic than tacrine. Phase II resulted in a statistically significant improvement in cognitive performance without drug-related liver effects, and Phase III trials have begun. (Incidentally, Shire worked on the clinical package for tacrine before passing it over to Warner-Lambert.)

Shire takes projects at various stages of development and progresses them through to early Phase III, then seeks partners from the major pharmaceutical companies (e.g. Janssen for galanthamine) for co-development and subsequent marketing in countries where it does not have a marketing presence. The costs of developing products to early Phase III (including the original cost of acquisition) are normally £3–4m, whereas Shire aim to recoup £5–7m in upfront payments and development contributions following a deal with a partner. In addition, the deal would include substantial royalties at a rate of

---

* Note added proof: Lafon has been reported to have left the Consortium 'to pursue different strategies'.

around 20%. The partner is necessary for the Shire's success, by providing access to global registration and marketing capabilities, in addition to bearing the bulk of the costs of late development.

In addition to the above major projects, Shire has other interests in off-patent products which are added value through formulation improvements or by other means, to extend the range or life-cycle of the product. Shire also operates a contract development division, which develops products for clients in return for a fee and perhaps a royalty share.

All toxicology and clinical trial work is contracted out, and the company has a collaboration with Chiroscience for the chiral synthesis of galanthamine. Shire's Chief Executive points to the virtual structure having advantages for its internal people, who are able to spend more time on planning and directing the company towards its strategic goals, rather than being diverted by operational management issues.

Despite a portfolio of about 7 major strategic projects and 13 tactical projects in development, in addition to others in registration or launched, Shire has spent modestly on R&D. From fiscal 1995 to 1996, expenditure rose substantially from £4.9m to £8.2m, largely due to galanthamine development. In 1996, the company floated on the London Stock Exchange, raising £21m for future investment. Its strategy of virtual integration has permitted internal costs to be kept to a minimum, and has generated a number of products which have allowed the company to become profitable within four years of being set up. The reasons behind this success owe a good deal to necessity, but it is also fair to say that the company has made this necessity into a virtue. Shire's turnover grew by 270% in 1995, and its marketing arm is now growing at a pace three times that of the UK industry average.

6.8   CONCLUSION

The changes in the traditional pharmaceutical industry since 1990 are profound and irreversible. The industry has shed 52 000 jobs as a result of 16 mergers from 1989 to 1996; this number will still increase as a result of decisions that have already been made but not yet fully implemented. Many of these losses will have been in research and development functions, which are necessary for the future of the industry. Despite the increased workload and stress felt by those who are left, the previous level of output is not possible with these reduced staffing levels. Moreover, the rapid advances that are occurring in some disciplines, and the need to acquire new technology that is likely to be of key importance for drug discovery, make the outsourcing of these functions of benefit for the industry as a whole. Therefore, to a certain extent, the traditional pharmaceutical industry needs to outsource increasing amounts of its R&D in order to bring new products to the market. The alternative option, to posit the decline of R&D as a requirement for the industry as a whole, is to ignore the long-term future in terms of products.

This argument points to a certain degree of permanence within the biotechnology sector and to growth in CROs. There are suggestions from some analysts that small companies will provide the major source of employment for new entrants into the pharmaceutical industry in the future. Certainly, companies such as Millennium, which has six long-term, lucrative collaborations with major pharmaceutical companies totalling $300m in value, of which $250m is committed, are likely to continue to grow. The principles underlying the prospects of companies like Millennium are for survival of the fittest, and failure in some measure for those that cannot perform. The vast and increasing array of options available in terms of provision of services leads to many different possibilities for the relationship between large company and provider. As far as provision of a component of the research or development process is concerned, one of the key issues is whether the relationship involves outsourcing the discovery process, including (some component of) the intellectual property rights. If it does, then clearly the acquisition of these rights involves some form of payment to the provider. The value of this commodity is contingent on the risky process of pharmaceutical R&D, and any small company whose existence is predicated upon royalty return on such discoveries—such as in terms of ability to raise money through stock offerings—is open to these risk elements. On the other hand, CROs which are traditionally not involved in discovery, and which are not liable to receive royalties on products that they develop, are reliant on a steadier, less risky but also less potentially lucrative income. Academic institutions involved in collaborations with industry are not generally analysed in this way because they are buffered by substantial public funding and are not commercial businesses. The issue of intellectual property rights normally defines the collaborative arrangements as being ones of partnership or of contract.

Although outsourcing is commonplace in other industries, the pharmaceutical industry is unusual in the breadth and depth of services that can be provided by this means. The peaks and troughs of drug research and development make it an ideal industry to utilise contractual services, and the extent to which it will do so in future shows every sign of increasing. The role of CROs in development, particularly in later developmental activities, is well established, but the most dramatic possibilities for outsourcing for the next few years lie in earlier development and research. There is substantial challenge in the management of such activities, because of the unpredictability of all research, but the principles of efficiency and economy, among others, apply to this phase as much as to later development.

The extent to which a company chooses to use external resources depends upon its particular circumstances and need within a certain project for the work to be done. Certain core operations may be best retained internally, because the expertise is there, even if the level of demand at peak times cannot be met and delays accrue. There is a spectrum of extent of outsourcing which may be adopted, from it being a minor activity to it being the main focus of operation. The varieties of strategies being adopted within the pharmaceutical industry are becoming more numerous with time.

Many of the virtual companies referred to in Chapter 6 have concentrated on the development of drugs rather than their research. Preclinical research bears a large proportion of the overall costs of bringing a new product to market, as was shown in Table 1.6, partly because of the high attrition rate in progressing through to market. The potential advantages (and disadvantages) for the virtual research or development company compared to the traditional self-contained mode of drug R&D nevertheless remain the same. Companies such as KS Biomedix and AMRAD are breaking new ground in forming relationships at early stages of research with academic institutes in efforts to commercialise their work. These are interesting developments, since a good deal of science of extremely high quality is conducted in academic institutions with insufficient contemplation, let alone development of commercial value.

The key attribute of the virtual company which sets it apart from the other ventures in the biotechnology sector is the low level of funding that seems to be required potentially to generate success. The figures reported above for the costs of development of new chemical entities will, if true, revolutionise the pharmaceutical industry. The traditional marketing requirement for the therapeutic target to be capable of commanding a peak sales return in excess of $150m per year will no longer be apparent. Rare diseases, and other markets in developing countries, can be considered, which hitherto have been disregarded. There will remain some diseases, and some economies, for which the pharmaceutical industry cannot make a return on its investment. But the level at which this consideration needs to be applied will be vastly different from today. If this concept becomes a widespread reality, rather than the embryonic idea it currently represents, it could provide a new framework for the provision of new medicines for society, and something akin to a miracle cure for the pharmaceutical industry.

References

1   Kunze ZM, Drasdo AL, Halliday RG and Lumley CE, 1993. Trends in worldwide pharmaceutical R&D. Expenditure for the 1990s. Centre for Medicines Research, Carshalton, Surrey, UK.

2   Brown PJ, 1995. Are companies masters of their own destinies? *Scrip Magazine*, April, 3.

3   Lendrem D, 1995. A clear case of more haste, less development speed. *Scrip Magazine*, December, 22.

4   Spilker B, 1989. *Multinational Drug Companies: Issues in Drug Discovery and Development*. Raven Press, New York.

5   Cox B, 1989. Strategies for drug discovery: structuring serendipity. *Pharm J*, **243**, 6551.

6   Martin YC, 1981. A practitioner's perspective of the role of quantitative structure-activity analysis in medicinal chemistry. *J Med Chem*, **24**, 229.

7   *Medicinal Chemistry: Principles and Practice*, 1994. Ed. FD King, Royal Society for Chemistry Press, Cambridge.

8   Cody RJ, 1994. The clinical potential of renin inhibitors. *Drugs*, **47**, 586.

9   Gallop MA, Barrett RW, Dower WJ, Fodor SPA and Gordon EA, 1994. Applications of combinatorial technologies to drug discovery. *J Med Chem*, **37**, 1233.

10 Terrett NK, Gardner M, Gordon DW, Koblecki RJ and Steel J, 1995. Combinatorial synthesis: the design of compound libraries and their application to drug discovery. *Tetrahedron*, **51**, 8135.

11 Ashton MJ, Jaye MC and Mason JS, 1996. New perspectives in lead generation II: evaluating molecular diversity. *Drug Discovery Today*, **1**, 71.

12 Manallack D, 1996. Getting that hit: 3D database searching in drug discovery. *Drug Discovery Today*, **1**, 231.

13 Brower V, 1994. Shaman—tapping in to tropical resources. *Scrip Magazine*, May, 53.

14 Lutz MW, Menius JA, Choi TD, Laskody RG, Domanico PL, Goetz AS and Saussy DL, 1996. Experimental design for high-throughput screening. *Drug Discovery Today*, **1**, 277.

15 Kilpatrick M, 1995. Manufacturing techniques in the service of drug discovery. *Scrip Magazine*, November, 6.

16　Cookson C, 1995. Technology: drugs that deliver. *Financial Times*, 28 September.
　　Bender LH, 1995. Drug delivery—a low risk path to better disease management. *Scrip Magazine*, November, 29.
17　Ankier SI and Warrington SJ, 1989. Research and development of new medicines. *J Int Med Res*, **17**, 407.
18　Polastro ET, 1995. Managing primary development for competitive edge. *Scrip Magazine*, November, 33.
19　Spilker B, 1995. Overview of medicines development. *Drug News and Perspectives*, April, 146.
20　Marty M, Pouillart P, Scholl S, Droz JP, Azab M, Brion N, Pujade-Lauraine E, Paule B, Paes D and Bons J, 1990. Comparison of the 5-hydroxytryptamine-3 (serotonin) antagonist ondansetron (GR38032F) with high dose metoclopromide in the control of cisplatin-induced emesis. *New Engl J Med*, **322**, 816.
　　Cunningham D, Pople A, Ford HT, Hawthorn J, Gazet J-C, Challoner T and Coombes RC, 1987. Prevention of emesis in patients receiving cytotoxic drugs by GR38032F, a selective 5-HT$_3$ receptor antagonist. *Lancet*, 27 June, 1461.
21　Oxford AW, Bell JA, Kilpatrick GA, Ireland SJ and Tyers MA, 1995. Ondansetron and related 5-HT$_3$ antagonists: recent advances. *Progr Med Chem*, **29**, 239.
22　Richardson BP, Engel G and Donatsch PA, 1985. Identification of serotonin M-receptor subtypes and their specific blockade by a new class of drugs. *Nature*, 316, 126.
23　Fozard JR and Gittos MW, 1983. Selective blockade of 5-hydroxytryptamine neuronal receptors by benzoic acid esters of tropine. *Brit J Pharmacol*, **80**, 511.
24　Tassignon J-P, 1995. Improving the drug development process. *Applied Clinical Trials*, **4**, 20.
25　(a) Herzog R, 1995. Project management: general aspects. *Drug News and Perspectives*, **7**, 486.
　　(b) Herzog R, 1995. Project management: pharmaceutical aspects. *Drug News and Perspectives*, **7**, 557.
　　(c) Herzog R, 1995. Project management: practical aspects. *Drug News and Perspectives*, **7**(10), 632.
26　Williams M and Malick JB, 1987. *Drug Discovery and Development*. Humana Press, New Jersey.
27　Wenzel AF, 1993. Von Wirkstoff zum Arzneimittel: F&E-Projektmanagement in der pharmazeutischen Industrie. *Projekt Management*, **3**, 4.
28　Data published on the World Wide Web at http://www.recap.com.
29　Grabowski H, 1991. Pharmaceutical research and development: returns and risk. Centre for Medicines Research Annual Lecture, Carshalton, Surrey, UK.
　　DiMasa JA, Hansen RW, Grabowski HG and Lasagna L, 1991. Cost of innovation in the pharmaceutical industry. *J Health Economics*, **10**, 107.
30　Prentis RA and Walker SR, 1985. Pharmaceutical research and development in the UK. *Pharm J*, 23 November, 676.
31　Lee KB and Hu LS, 1996. Biotechnology: past, present and future. *Chem Ind*, 6 May, 334.
32　Pharma Pipelines, 1996. Lehman Brothers, London.

33 *Pharmaceutical Business News*, 1996. FDA approval progress: agency and PhRMA conflict, 31 January, 17.
34 Lumley C and Walker S, 1995. Improving the regulatory review process. Centre for Medicines Research, Carshalton, Surrey, UK.
35 Schwartz H, 1996. Buchanan and the pharmaceutical industry. *Scrip*, 2107, 16.
36 Hill T and Hubbard J, 1996. Is outsourcing clinical trials really more expensive? *Scrip Magazine*, March, 19.
37 Drews J, 1995. The impact of cost containment on pharmaceutical research and development. CMR Annual Lecture, Carshalton, Surrey, UK.
38 Roberts I, 1994. Evaluating R&D investments. *Scrip Magazine*, November, 16.
39 Roberts I, 1995. Financial analysis of licensing opportunities. *Drug News and Perspectives*, **8**(8), 509.
40 Weiss M, Nick M and Opsetmoen K, 1995. Cash flows and the strategic management of risk. *Scrip Magazine*, June, 10.
41 Johnson G, 1996. What place for R&D in tomorrow's drug industry? *Drug Discovery Today*, **1**(3), 117.
42 Poste G, 1996. The human genome project: implications for the future of the pharmaceutical industry. Centre for Medicines Research Annual Lecture, Carshalton, Surrey, UK.
43 Page CP, Sutter MC and Walker MJA, 1994. Wither, whether and whither pharmacology. *Trends Pharmacol Sci*, **15**, 17.
44 Employee Selection in the UK, 1988. Institute for Manpower Studies, Sussex, UK.
45 Drews J, 1992. Strategies for successfully managing pharmaceutical research and development in the 1990s. *Drug Information Journal*, **26**(4), 635.
46 Burke M, 1994. Transfusing the lifeblood of the industry. *Chemistry and Industry*, 18 July, 548.
47 Evans P, 1996. Streamlining formal portfolio management. *Scrip Magazine*, February, 25.
48 Duplantier AJ and Turner CR, 1996. Novel pharmacological approaches to the treatment of asthma: status and potential of therapeutic classes. *Drug Discovery Today*, **1**, 199.
49 Wade N, 1981. *The Nobel Duel*. Anchor Press/Doubleday, New York.
50 Arnold R and Grindley J, 1996. Matchmaking: identifying and evaluating drug discovery partners. *Drug Discovery Today*, **1**, 79.
51 Hovde M, 1995. Choosing and using CROs. *Scrip Magazine*, July/August, 28.
52 *The Technomark Register of CROs in Europe*, 1995. Talentmark, London.
53 *Soteros Directory of Non-clinical Research and Consultancy Services*, 1995. Soteros Consultants Limited, Huntingdon, UK.
54 *The Directory of University Expertise and Facilities: Biosciences*, 1994/5. Oakland Consultancy, Cambridge, UK.
55 Blumenthal D, Causino N, Campbell E and Louis KS, 1996. Relationships between academic institutions and industry in the life sciences. *New Engl J Med*, **334**, 368.
56 Herzog R, 1995. Managing international R&D. *Drug News and Perspectives*, **8**(3), 177.

57   Taylor P, 1995. Innovation networking—a driving force in R&D. *Scrip Magazine*, July/August, 42.
58   Welch AD, 1985. Reminiscences in pharmacology: auld acquaintances ne'er forgot. *Annu Rev Pharmacol Toxicol*, **25**, 1.
59   Cushman DW and Ondetti MA, 1980. Inhibitor of angiotensin converting enzyme. *Prog Med Chem*, **17**, 42.
60   Kenney M, 1986. *The University–Industrial Complex*. Yale University Press, New Haven and London.
61   Konecny E, Quinn CP, Sachs K and Thompson DT, 1995. *Universities and Industrial Research*. The Royal Society of Chemistry, Cambridge, UK.
62   Mowery DC and Rosenberg N, 1989. *Technology and the Pursuit of Economic Growth*. Cambridge University Press, Cambridge, UK.
63   Kealey GTE, 1996. *The Economic Laws of Science*. Macmillan Press, London.
64   HMSO, 1993. Realising our potential: a strategy for science. *Engineering and Technology*, London.
65   Johnson G, 1994. *University Politics*. Cambridge University Press, Cambridge, UK.
66   Persidis A, Dunn III WE and MacMillan IC, 1996. Parascientific training for PhDs. *Nature Biotechnology*, **14**, 406.
67   Shohet S and Prevezer M, 1996. UK biotechnology: institutional linkages, technology transfer and the role of intermediaries. *R&D Management*, **26**(3), 283.
68   Senker P and Senker J, 1994. Transferring technology and expertise from universities to industry: Britain's teaching company scheme. *New Technology, Work and Employment*, **9**, 81.
69   Thomas D, 1995. Innovate to survive. *Chemistry and Industry*, 4 December, 973.
70   Webster A and Swain V, 1991. The pharmaceutical industry: towards a new innovation environment. *Technology Analysis and Strategic Management*, **3**, 127.
71   Sullivan NF, 1995. *Technology Transfer*. Cambridge University Press, Cambridge, UK.
72   Rappert B, 1995. Shifting notions of accountability in public- and private-sector research in the UK: some central concerns. *Science and Public Policy*, **22**, 383.
73   Flack JD, 1986. Toxicity: ritual, rational and regulatory requirements. In *Prediction and Assessment of Antibiotic Clinical Efficacy*, Ed. FO Grady and A Percival. Academic Press, London and Orlando.
74   Brown D, 1995. Accelerating drug development without increasing risk. *Insight*, Issue 2, 59.
75   Balls MPA, Botham LH, Brunter and Spielmann H, 1995. The EC/HO International Validation Study on Alternatives to the Draize Eye Irritation Test. *Toxicology in vitro*, **9**, 871–929.
76   Drug discovery on the fast track, 1995. *Pharma Business*, Sep/Oct, 54.
77   Moses E and Brimblecombe R, 1995. Bridging the technology gap. *Scrip Magazine*, July/August, 8.
78   *European Biotech 96: Volatility and Value*. Ernst & Young, London.
79   Cavalla D, 1996. Has chirality been oversold? *Scrip Magazine*, 3 March, 13.
80   Hartley D, 1995. Accelerating Products to Clinical Evaluation. *IBC*

Symposium on Pharmaceutical Pre-Clinical Development, Le Meridien, London, 4–5 December.

81 Rees P, 1996. Combinatorial chemistry solutions for the desktop. *Scientific Computing World*, February, 25.

82 Wallace BM and Lasker JS, 1993. *Science*, **250**, 912.

83 Bodor N, Prokai L, Wu W-M, Farag H, Jonalagadda S, Kawamura M and Simpkins J, 1992. A strategy for delivering peptides into the central nervous system by sequential metabolism. *Science*, **257**, 1698.

84 Drews J, 1995. Future prospects for the pharmaceutical industry. *Pharmaceutical Manufacturing*, **25**.

85 Mark R and Clark WW, 1984. Gothic structural experimentation. *Scientific American*, **251**, 144.

86 Lawrence S and Harvey C, 1995. *Scrip Magazine*, April, 11.

87 Steiner J, 1995. The reality of virtuality in drug development. *Scrip Magazine*, December, 24.

88 Shaw B, 1995. Looking for a lead in IT. *Scrip Magazine*, October, 21.

89 Todtling F, 1994. Regional networks of high-technology firms—the case of the Greater Boston area. *Technovation*, **14**, 342.

90 Hughes D, 1996. Controlling proliferation through collaboration. *Drug Discovery Today*, **1**, 405.

91 Byrne JA, Brandt R and Port O, 1993. The virtual corporation. *Business Week*, 8 February, 103.

Index

Index compiled by Liza Weinkove